Hugh Miller has written many books of non-fiction and several novels including the bestsellers *Ambulance*, *The Dissector*, *Silent Witnesses* and *Casualty*. He is an acknowledged expert on forensic medicine and has many TV credits including *Emmerdale* and *EastEnders*. His recent crime novels featuring charismatic detective Mike Fletcher drew consistently high praise from reviewers on both sides of the Atlantic.

pg. 176-177 — true sadomasic. vs fetish people

pg. 177-178 — sex offenders cannot be "treated"

pg. 223-224 — More on the BS psychiatrists sling on behalf of criminals

Unquiet Minds

The World of
Forensic Psychiatry

Hugh Miller

HEADLINE

First published in 1994
by HEADLINE BOOK PUBLISHING

First published in paperback in 1995
by HEADLINE BOOK PUBLISHING

10 9 8 7 6 5 4 3 2

ISBN 0 7472 4646 7

Phototypeset by Intype, London
Printed and bound in Great Britain by
Cox & Wyman Ltd, Reading, Berkshire

HEADLINE BOOK PUBLISHING
A division of Hodder Headline PLC
338 Euston Road
London NW1 3BH

Contents

Acknowledgements

Doctors are rarely comfortable about being named in connection with the critical or the controversial. 'Quote me but don't identify me,' is a stricture I lived with when I was writing *Casualty* and, a couple of years later, *Silent Witnesses*. I heard it several times during the preparation of this book, too. In a time of universal volubility, such reticence on the part of medical people is still understandable, given the rules of conduct by which they are muzzled. Wherever I was asked, I have respected their wishes and changed the names of a number of doctors quoted in the text.

The benevolence of medical professionals works in inverse ratio to their longing for publicity. Forensic psychiatrists proved to be especially generous: I can't remember when I was ever so kindly accommodated, or so painstakingly helped. For case material, anecdotes, guidance and for so much else, I am indebted and grateful to an exact dozen individuals in Europe and the United States.

One consultant psychiatrist, in particular, lightened the

work. Dr Elaine Edmunds was unstinting with her advice in the preparation and editing of the case notes, and with her time and instructive comments during a critical reading of the chapters. Whatever virtues of accuracy and relevance the book has, they would have been fewer without her support.

Preface

Forensic psychiatry had its origins in the last century, but its evolution as a speciality in the United Kingdom did not get under way until some time in the middle-to-late 1960s. Over the years it has attracted little attention to itself, it has been described by the World Health Organisation as 'an ill-defined speciality', and as yet the majority of people are vague about what forensic psychiatrists are or what they do. So, a brief explanation may not be out of place.

Forensic psychiatrists are involved at every point where the law and psychiatry touch or overlap, although in practice they are mainly engaged in dealing with mentally disordered offenders. The responsibilities of the profession call for a sound working knowledge of the law, civil and criminal. Practitioners are also required to determine a defendant's level of responsibility, to evaluate his fitness for trial – no matter how much bluffing is going on – and to produce a detailed and coherent psychiatric court report. They also decide such things as testamentary capacity (the ability to make a will), and violent lawbreakers' varying levels of dangerousness.

'I was a real blue-eyed virgin when I started dealing with offenders,' said Judith, now a seasoned forensic psychiatrist. 'But it didn't take long to find out what devious swine a lot of them are. I've met some who actually study mental illness. They watch psychiatric patients who've been released into the community, and they pick up pointers. In fifteen years of practice I've come across some magnificent actors, men and women and even children, simulating all shades of psychosis, and giving it everything they've got.'

She remembered a woman defendant in a theft case taking a glass test tube from her pocket and calmly eating it. An emergency washout was performed and a note went on the record to indicate that the woman was mentally disturbed. But months later the same patient tried the same trick with another psychiatrist.

'And that's what it was,' Judith said, 'a trick. A bit of intensive questioning and some background inquiry uncovered the fact that her former husband, a circus performer, had taught her how to do that and lots of other unpleasant stunts.'

Other imaginative offenders have thrown fits during psychiatric interviews, they have talked psychotic gibberish, gone into impressive trances and even spontaneously bled from the ears.

'Time has blessed me with a touch of wisdom and a lot of suspicion,' Judith said. 'Spotting fakers is a challenge which I take very personally. I never let myself forget I'm working in the muddy territory between madness and badness. I stay alert all the time. These days they have to be pretty good to get past me.'

Not every seemingly disturbed offender is faking. Most of them are not. But even when there is evidence of disturbance, a problem can arise when the psychiatrist won't be tied to a precise opinion of what is wrong. Such reluctance is not new, nor is it rare. Psychiatry is not, after all, a precise science; in the opinion of some people it is closer to astrology or witchcraft than it is to medicine, but that aside, it is often difficult to make an objective, sharp-edged decision where the criteria are so mutable. Because of the force of circumstances, some psychiatrists have made a craft out of indecision. As Dr Anthony Clare wrote some years ago,

> *Psychiatry . . . is fluid and uncertain, its practitioners have a penchant for ambivalence and a tendency to avoid definitive statements save, it sometimes seems, when they cannot be backed up with supportive evidence!*

But often, even when the forensic psychiatrist decides a mental disorder is real, and is supported by evidence, and has a name, there are other psychiatrists ready to say the patient is shamming, or that the so-called disorder does not exist. A number of recurring disagreements are aired within the cases in the following pages. The main areas of friction appear to be a belief on one side that all crime, to some extent, is a manifestation of mental disturbance, and the opposing certainty that many people are just plain bad and should be punished for it.

This book is not primarily about forensic psychiatry, but about the cases encountered by its practitioners. These are real cases, taken directly from the files of practising psychiatrists, and published here for the first time. They are intended for study and discussion by both laymen and professionals. Many cases make grim and uncomfortable reading; at times it seems that no light has touched the overcast reaches of the human mind since the Middle Ages. A tribute to the dogged objectivity of doctors and police officers is the fact that such extremes of chaos, of horror and spiritual agony can be refined to cool disquisition and clear argument, fit to enter the legal process.

Among accounts of crimes and outrages spawned by unbalanced minds, the reader will find instances of cool-headed, calculated wickedness committed by terribly sane people. Such histories tend to demonstrate, as if further demonstration were needed, that greed and compulsive spite make man the most implacably vicious creature extant.

'It's sadly true that people are driven to damage anything helpless,' said Judith. 'That's at the heart of so much crime we see, whether the perpetrator's mentally disturbed or completely sane.'

She does not believe her profession can do anything to change that.

'We help to arrest trends, and we sometimes forestall them before they get under way,' she said. 'We make sure some dangerous people are kept from harming the public, and we defuse the danger in others. On balance, I would say we justify our existence. But even at our best, I suppose we're no better than tiny lights in a terrible dark place.'

Hugh Miller
Warwick, June 1994

1
Sadistic Personality

Among psychiatrists, especially the ones who define the categories of mental illness and decide on the terminology to be used to describe the various ailments, Sadistic Personality Disorder is a controversial diagnosis. Some criticise it because they do not believe the condition exists as a distinct psychiatric disorder; others believe it does exist, but they cannot agree on its diagnostic features.

Broadly speaking, Sadistic Personality Disorder is the name given to a pervasive, persistent pattern of behaviour where a person takes pleasure in being cruel and physically violent towards other people. He or she is often fascinated by violence and by the various ways to inflict pain, and will in many cases take pleasure in the mental agony induced by fear both in human beings and animals.

A German specialist, who made detailed studies of over a hundred cases in an eleven-year period, said she could sum up the majority of Sadistic Personality Disorders in a handful of prominent traits which they all seem to share to varying degrees.

'A bit of assiduous probing usually uncovers the fact that they have used physical violence or cruelty as a means of taking control of a relationship,' she said. 'They are absolutely *besotted* with the practice of humiliating their partners, or other close persons, in the presence of others.'

In their attitude to animals, she said, people with Sadistic Personality Disorder usually gave her the impression that they did not really believe the creatures had much purpose or value, and that it was quite in order to find pleasure in hurting them.

'They compulsively restrict the independence of people to whom they are close – lovers, spouses – usually by refusing to let them do anything on their own or go anywhere alone, or with other friends. And they will, as a matter of routine, lie or cheat or create mischief in some way, to cause harm to those they purport to love, or for whom they profess some feeling of closeness.'

Invariably, she said, their fascination with violence and the instruments of injury goes far beyond the range of normal curiosity or enthusiasm.

The first of the following cases has been described as a classic illustration of Sadistic Personality Disorder coupled with Antisocial Personality Disorder.

CASE ONE: *The Search for Perfection*

In October 1979 Dieter Frink, thirty-two, described in the tabloid press at the time of his arrest as 'coarse and degenerate looking', was charged in München with the homicides of ten women over an eight-week period. The murders were the culmination of a long, grotesque criminal career which had its roots in Frink's childhood in a poor southern suburb of Berlin.

Giving evidence at Frink's trial, a criminologist put emphasis on the fact that the prisoner had been brutally treated as a child, and suggested he might not have led such a downgrade adult life if his childhood had been even slightly touched by the accepted standards of protection and care. A forensic psychiatrist and a clinical psychologist went further: they put forward the view that Frink would have grown into an ordinary conforming adult, with no special abnormalities in his behaviour, had it not been for his bizarre upbringing.

'Beneath the grossness and depravity infesting every level of the defendant's view of life,' said the psychiatrist, 'there are lingering traces of normal human impulses and humane response mechanisms – in other words an actual set of decent human values, but they have been crippled and repressed by the hideous circumstances of his treatment as a child.'

Hans Kuchelmann, a specialist in criminal psychology, read a newspaper report of the trial and wrote to the *Jahrbuch der Psychiatrie* to complain that the court was being misled by sentimental, wrong-headed assessments of a man who was clearly bad and would never have been any better, whatever the circumstances of his childhood.

It is perfectly clear to anyone in day-to-day contact with criminals, he wrote, *that certain individuals are structured to work against the prevailing morality. They are equipped with contrary instincts, and so deviation and subversion are the characteristics of such persons, just as kindness and good humour may be outstanding characteristics of others. In-built features of a person's character should never be mistaken for distortions brought about by environment or upbringing. Such dis-*

*tortions exist, of course, but they are never so prominent
or extreme as the vicious impulses and repugnant
psychosexual traits exhibited by the defendant in this
case. Dieter Frink is not a sick man, he is a bad man.
There is no cure for his behaviour because it is not a
sickness, and he should not be represented to the jury
as a victim, when in fact he is decidedly a cold-blooded
victimiser on whom sympathy and compassion would
be wasted.*

Professor Kuchelmann's views were never presented to the
court and were not published until after Frink's trial, but a
police witness called by the prosecution did put forward
a similar view in open court. When he was asked if he had
ever come across anyone like Dieter Frink before, the officer said he never had.

'I have met men who have murdered children, and men
who killed other people for money, but none of them were
as cold as Frink. He gives the feeling that he's completely
heartless, in fact not quite human.'

The officer was asked whether, in his experience of dealing with people, he could identify Frink as being a man in
need of any kind of help.

'He's not sick, if that's what you're asking,' the officer
said. 'The sickness is in anybody who would believe that
kind of garbage.'

Dieter Frink was raised as the youngest of five children.
He was born at a time when his mother Anna, an alcoholic,
was being divorced by her husband because of her drunken-
ness and habitual adultery. From the earliest time Dieter
could remember, Anna blamed him for the fact she had no
husband and therefore no regular source of support.

'She told me if she hadn't been carrying me, he would never have divorced her at all. The pregnancy was the whole reason for the marriage breaking up.'

Anna's resentment of the child was intensified by the fact that three attempts at abortion, one of which nearly killed her, had no effect on the foetus. 'You wouldn't budge, you little bastard . . .'

Dieter's biological father was a married janitor from a nearby sports gymnasium who committed suicide when Dieter was two years old. Following the janitor's death his widow made numerous attempts to attack Dieter's mother, both on the street and at home. On one occasion she threw a glassful of spirits of salt (hydrochloric acid) through an open window, narrowly missing Anna's eyes. From that time, according to one of Dieter's sisters, Anna set her heart even harder against the boy, blaming him for every misfortune she suffered, even claiming that he was the reason she could not kick her drinking habit.

Anna routinely beat the boy, and even before he was able to walk she had begun to torture him. X-rays taken when he was an adult showed that two fingers on his right hand and one on his left had been fractured in infancy. More than twenty years later he could recall the intense pain as Anna twisted the joints until they broke.

'She knew things like that, about hurting kids,' Dieter's sister told the forensic psychiatrist. 'One of the boyfriends used to talk to her about it, about how kids would feel more pain in their fingers than anywhere else, or how they wouldn't make a noise when you were hitting them if you pushed a pencil or something else hard into their anus. She was a cruel mother, but she learned it all off other people.'

Dieter told the same psychiatrist that when he was two or three years old, his mother used to pull hairs out of his head one at a time. 'Sometimes I'd be falling asleep and I would wake up suddenly with the pain. Then she would hit me for crying, and bawl at me for not sleeping at night like the other kids.'

Anna had regular lovers, usually other alcoholics, some of whom lived with her for months at a stretch. She encouraged these men to call Dieter 'little Pissy', because of his habit of bed-wetting, which persisted from infancy through to his early adult years. From the age of approximately five, Dieter's punishment for bed-wetting was to stand by an open window with the wet sheet draped over his head until it was dried by the breeze. An alternative punishment was to make him go for an entire day without anything to drink.

One of Anna's men friends, a truck driver who often stayed with her at weekends, developed a strong dislike for her children, and for Dieter in particular.

'He used to urinate in a milk bottle and make me drink it,' Dieter said. 'He quite often burned me on the hands and arms with his cigar, too, and when he got really drunk he would make my sisters do sex with him.'

After a time Anna actively joined in the abuse of her children. She later told Dieter that she had done it because she was afraid the man would beat her if she did not. During the psychiatric evaluation, Dieter revealed that for years, his mother had been the object of his most intense sexual fantasy.

'I imagined hanging her up by the feet, then cutting her clothes off her with a razor. Then I'd make cuts all over her body and watch the blood run out and join up in streams that would drip off her head on to the floor. Sometimes I still think about hanging her up in the closet, spraying her all over with rubbing alcohol then lighting her up . . .'

Dieter began committing burglaries with another boy when he was seven. He was small and thin and could easily squeeze through cat flaps and other small spaces, but although he regularly stole cameras, jewellery and other valuable items, there was very little profit in the venture.

'The people we tried to sell the stuff to, most of them would just take it off us, and if we made a noise about it they would hit us, or threaten to get the law.'

At the age of twelve Dieter was caught raiding a pharmacy and was put on probation. A year later he was sent to a youth corrective centre for committing 'lewd and lascivious acts' with a six-year-old girl.

'The correction centre was the worst place I've been in, ever,' he told the forensic psychiatrist. 'Anything I did was wrong. I got beaten nearly every day. They did it with wet towels, or with pillowcases filled with oranges, things that really hurt but didn't make any deep marks, or hardly any.'

In the correction centre Dieter was sodomised by other inmates. As a result of a particularly brutal assault by three youths in their late teens, his anus was torn and he became seriously ill with septicaemia. He spent three weeks in the infirmary. On the day he was released and sent back to his room at the centre, he was sodomised again by two older inmates.

Between the ages of fourteen and seventeen he faced a number of charges of armed robbery and car theft; although he was probably guilty in every instance, his luck held to the extent that there was never enough evidence to allow the police to take the charges forward to prosecution. He admitted to the forensic psychiatrist that he believed he had killed another boy when he was fourteen.

'For some reason I didn't like him, it could make me mad just looking at him. One night we were by the canal near where I lived, and I argued with him about something, and before I knew it I'd shot him with a little Mauser I used to have. He fell into the canal. I waited but he never came up. So for a while after that I kept my ears open, waiting to hear he'd been found, but he never was. His mother was sure he had run away, and so that was it, over and done with. I've no idea what really happened to him, but I'm pretty sure I did kill him.'

At the age of seventeen Dieter married for the first time. The girl was Magda, twenty-two, a self-styled beautician with a record of soliciting and drug dealing. The marriage lasted two years and during that time the couple produced a daughter, Maria. When the child was a little over a year old, Dieter caught Magda in bed with another woman. He beat her savagely and she ran away from home, taking the child with her. Three months later Magda's dead body was found in a cheap lodging house in Tutzing. The child was in bed beside the corpse, trying to feed it chocolate. An autopsy disclosed that Magda had died of an overdose of barbiturates. The little girl, Maria, was put in the protective care of her maternal grandmother, although Dieter managed to get visiting rights.

Over a period of fourteen years Dieter married seven times in all. From the age of sixteen he had entertained a growing fantasy of finding the perfect woman; his idea was that when he found her he would marry her and be happy for the rest of his life. His notion of female perfection was eternal desirability – he wanted to find a woman who would so excite him sexually that he would never tire of her. Several times he believed he had located the perfect partner, but the illusion never lasted long. He always ended up beating his wives and girlfriends, some of them seriously, and most of the marriages lasted no more than a few months. When one wife told him she wanted out of the marriage, he responded by beating up her parents.

Following a series of armed hold-ups at liquor stores and supermarkets, Dieter was sentenced, at the age of twenty-four, to five years' imprisonment. While he was in prison he embarked on a career of 'protection' with two other men. He was implicated in the death of a prisoner who appeared to have been thrown from a laundry roof, but no charges were brought. Late in the second year of his prison sentence, Dieter molested his six-year-old daughter during a conjugal visit.

He served three-and-a-half years in prison. When he was released he lived for a time with his mother – she was now suffering from leukaemia – at her small flat in Bremen. While he was living there he impregnated a forty-year-old woman, a friend of his mother, who eventually reported him to the police for breaking her arm because she refused to submit to anal intercourse. The court ordered that Dieter be placed in an institution where he would undertake psychiatric treatment for what the magistrates called his 'chronic and seemingly psychotic aggression'.

The superintendent of the institution, a behavioural psychologist of the old school, was not happy about having such a disruptive influence about the place, but he had no option. He was ordered to accept Dieter for treatment.

'I found him rather a frightening man,' the superintendent told journalists years later. 'He could go through the motions of civilised behaviour and even display a quite sunny disposition, but it was obvious he was wearing the appearance and behaviour as a disguise. You only had to look at his eyes and see the deadness in them to know he was a complete sociopath. He was always on the sidelines, watching, and only ever pretending to be one of the team. Once when he was alone with me, he told me he could kill me and make it look like an accident. He told me that clean out of the blue, when we were talking about something entirely different. When I told him rather hastily that I always carried a personal alarm, he smiled and told me it was only a joke, and not to take things so seriously.'

Therapy at the institution consisted mainly of light sedation and free-association conversational sessions with therapists and other patients. It appeared to do Dieter some good (although the superintendent probably gave him good ratings to get rid of him) and he was released a month earlier than scheduled. He celebrated his release by robbing a small supermarket, picking up two girls and spending twenty-four hours in bed with them.

After drifting for several years Dieter took up residence with his daughter Maria – now thirteen – after applying to a court for her custody, and finding it surprisingly easy to obtain. Custody was granted on the grounds that a parent, even one with a criminal record, was better able to supervise a teenage child than a semi-senile, alcoholic grandparent.

Dieter soon impregnated his daughter, and she had an abortion. For the next six years he assaulted the girl sexually at least once a week, and she had three further abortions. Once, when Dieter had hurt his foot and was not able to earn money by the usual criminal means, he forced Maria to have sex with three men in the space of an hour so that he would have cash to go out drinking. A few weeks later, when a friend of Maria's arrived for a two-week visit, Dieter raped her.

Maria finally informed the authorities about the six years of abuse. Felony charges were filed against Dieter for incest, unlawful sexual acts, sodomy and oral copulation. He responded by changing his name and moving to another town while he was on bail. Shortly after that he met a twenty-year-old girl who owned her own apartment and a customised camper van. He married her and two months later embarked on the series of murders for which he was subsequently imprisoned for life.

His new wife, Erika, who eventually testified against him, worked as his partner. She lured all but one of the victims to their deaths. Emotionally Erika was an incredibly passive young woman, keen to further her husband's fantasy of finding the 'perfect lover', and displaying no outward signs of jealousy or even mild distress. It transpired that she had no real capacity for loyalty, either, and could easily switch her allegiance to whoever impressed her at a particular time.

The first murder took place after Dieter picked up a girl called Ida in a town-centre bar and took her back to the apartment. Erika was in bed asleep. Ida had consumed nearly a whole bottle of rum and at the apartment she had three glasses of whisky while she and Dieter danced to taped music.

By the time they began to make love she was very drunk. During intercourse on the living-room floor she rolled on top of Dieter, stiffened suddenly and vomited in his face.

The incident sobered both of them. They cleaned up in the bathroom, and while Ida sat in a fireside chair smoking a cigarette and complaining of pains in her stomach, Dieter went to the kitchen and fetched a hammer. He hit her on top of the skull with it, twenty or thirty times, not stopping until her head was unrecognisable. By then the living room walls, doors and carpet were splashed profusely with blood.

Dieter woke Erika and explained what had happened.

Between them they rolled the body up in the polythene anti-frost cover they kept for the van. They spent three hours cleaning the walls and chopping the carpet into hundreds of small pieces, which Dieter packed into four large rubbish bags.

Finally, thick adhesive tape was wound around the polythene sheet covering the body, then Dieter drove it with the bags of chopped carpet to the municipal incinerator. He was able to push everything down the chute and into the flames without being challenged, or even raising the slightest official curiosity.

When he got back home he made love to Erika on the bare floorboards. Afterwards she listened to his detailed plans. Although his simple notion of perfection remained unchanged, his plans were stripped to essentials and had become chillingly more practical: prospects would be forced to have sex with him, and those who failed to show promise would be killed. Erika readily agreed to be his accomplice, showing no revulsion or even a trace of worry at the possibility of being implicated in serial murder.

Over the following two months the couple visited shopping centres and town and village fairs all over southern Germany. Erika appeared to take to her role easily. She accosted young girls who fitted Dieter's specification, talked them into climbing into the customised van, usually on the pretext of looking at 'hot' merchandise being offered at bargain prices. Once inside, the victims were confronted by Dieter, who held a handgun on them while Erika bound them with adhesive tape. She then climbed through to the front of the van and watched a video on a portable unit, while Dieter raped the victim, then shot or strangled her.

'Nobody ever refused me, or even tried to resist,' Erika told the police. 'I would just look for the right type, walk up to her and say what Dieter had told me to say, and the girl would come with me. Every time. I think people just trust me on sight.'

Most of the victims were petite blondes who looked like Erika, who in turn strongly resembled Dieter's daughter, Maria. Dieter had a rating system for each victim, and always made sure that Erika knew she was never Number One. If a victim struggled too much when he assaulted her, or for some other reason distracted him, he would fail to reach climax. When that happened, Dieter invariably killed the girl, then had intercourse with the body, at which time he would have no difficulty achieving an orgasm.

'I knew after the third or fourth one that he was always going to kill them,' Erika told the police. 'He stopped pretending he was looking for the perfect girl. Either that or he just dropped the idea. Killing them was the big kick, and knowing what would happen was part of the kick. He talked about it. When he got drunk, he told me, he liked to see a girl climbing into the van, all bright and curious, and him knowing that in just a little while he would have screwed her and she would be dead. It was the biggest turn-on ever.'

The bodies of the victims were buried at various sites across an area of fifty square kilometres. The police were first alerted to foul play when the naked, partially decomposed body of a young woman was found by a man whose dog would not stop digging at the base of a wall outside an electricity sub-station. Police were able to identify the woman as an art student who had been missing from her college residency for more than a month. Ligature marks around her neck suggested she had been strangled.

While the post-mortem examination was taking place, a report of another body being found came in from a police mobile patrol. They had been flagged down by a jogger who had seen a human foot protruding from a hillock of rubbish on a domestic-waste site. This finding turned out to be the body of Greta Sokel, nineteen, a laboratory assistant who had last been seen getting into a van parked on a side street at a market near the town of Starnberg.

At this point police records helped to short-cut what might otherwise have been a lengthy investigation. Details of a van fitting the description given by the witness had been routinely filed when, on the day Greta Sokel disappeared, the vehicle travelled the wrong way along a one-way street on the outskirts of Starnberg and was photographed by an automatic traffic camera. The photograph not only recorded the van's registration number, but clearly showed the face of the driver and the woman sitting beside him.

Dieter and Erika Frink were picked up within three hours of their van being identified. Frink's horrendous criminal record alerted the police to the possibility that this might become a major investigation. They immediately put the couple in different rooms and interviewed them separately. Erika was promised full immunity from prosecution if she would cooperate. She agreed to tell the police anything they wanted to know, and she was as good as her word. She even provided details of where the remaining eight bodies were to be found, including the one that had gone into the incinerator.

The trial of Dieter Frink lasted three weeks. When the judge finally sent the jury away to make their deliberations, he asked them to try to set aside their natural revulsion and concentrate wholly on the issues of law in the case. It was certainly not the hardest case to understand. The prosecution maintained that Dieter had murdered ten women, and they had provided powerful evidence to suggest that he certainly had. In Dieter's defence, his lawyers and expert witnesses had offered only the evidence of his terrible childhood, since there was no believable way to claim that he hadn't committed the murders, especially when Erika's testimony had been so clear and plausible.

Frink was found guilty of all ten murders, and the jury made no recommendation for mercy. He was sentenced to life imprisonment, with the stipulation that he should never be considered for parole.

CASE TWO: *Just a Beast . . .*
In October 1988 Derek Lewis, thirty-seven, was arrested at his home in Macclesfield, Cheshire, following a disturbance in which a neighbour, a woman in her twenties, was thrown from a bedroom window and suffered multiple injuries, including a broken neck. When Lewis's wife and three children were interviewed, it became clear that the police had stumbled on a sickening case of protracted cruelty. For four years Derek Lewis had sadistically beaten and sexually abused his own children and six more from another family.

'It was one of those catalogues you think is never going to stop,' a female psychiatrist said. 'One emetic fact led to another, and there were so many kids involved that the permutations of cruelty and obscenity seemed endless. We spoke with five of the children involved in the case, and with Lewis's wife and the woman he threw out of the window. The more they told us, the blacker the story became.'

The story pieced together by the psychiatrist and two of her colleagues showed that Derek Lewis had probably been overtly sadistic since he was in his early teens. He had first been in trouble with the police at thirteen for minor

offences – trespass and petty theft. When he was fourteen
he was judged to be 'in need of care and attention' and
was moved from the family home, where both parents were
alcoholics, and put in the care of the local authority. While
in the children's home he was reported for cutting the feet
off a budgerigar with scissors, and on another occasion he
dipped a live kitten in paraffin and set it on fire.

Lewis reached adulthood with a string of convictions
for petty offences behind him. He had a very fine talent for
wood-turning, and in his early twenties he made a respectable living selling hand-turned vases, lamp bases, fruit bowls
and egg cups to small exclusive shops on a contract basis.
During this period he married Eileen, a shop assistant, and
they set up home with her parents in their council house.

'That didn't work too well,' Eileen told a psychiatrist.
'My Dad was a stickler for tidiness and Derek wasn't. He
was dead casual about where he put stuff and how he left
things, and it got on Dad's nerves. He told Derek about it,
and at first Derek said OK, he was sorry, he would be a bit
tidier in future. But he wasn't, he just went on leaving his
things lying about in the kitchen and the living room, doing
wood-turning in Dad's shed and leaving the place like a
tip, until Dad exploded at him and said he could either
change his ways, or change his address. Derek fumed for
about an hour after that, sitting in our room, staring out
the window, then all at once he shot up, grabbed a walking
stick he'd been making for a special order, a real heavy big
thing, and he went downstairs and he hammered my Dad
with it. Put him in hospital with broken ribs and concussion,
and got himself three months for his trouble.'

Eileen had their first child, a boy, six months after they
moved into a rented flat at Gurnett. Derek had grown

bored with the steady routine of wood-turning for a living, and even though the money was good and he had no immediate alternative, he decided he would not do it any more. When Eileen complained that they would have no income, just at a time when they needed a bit extra, Derek took a sledgehammer round to his workshop, behind a neighbouring pub, and smashed his lathe with it. He then went into the pub and got very drunk. When he returned he forced Eileen to have sex with him, even though she still had painful stitches following the birth of the baby. She believed that as she lay on the floor afterwards, weeping with pain, Derek slapped the two-week-old baby because he was crying.

'At that time, it was like we went through a door or something,' Eileen said. 'A door into a dark place. Honest to God, I can't remember Derek ever being happy from the time the first baby was born. I can't think of a week after that when he didn't hit me, either.'

As the years passed Derek drifted in and out of one job after another, none of them skilled or particularly well paid. Two more children were born, a girl and a boy, and Eileen had to undergo a therapeutic abortion of a fourth pregnancy; the operation left her sterile, a fact she accepted with relief. Eventually the family moved into council accommodation in Macclesfield, and for a time Derek seemed to brighten. He even talked about going into business again on his own, but in spite of coaxing from Eileen he would not go back to wood-turning.

In 1984 he served a six-month prison term for assault on a child welfare officer. When he came out of prison he refused to work. He took control of the Family Allowance book and most of the other state benefits coming into the house. He spent the money on drink and gambling, and when Eileen pleaded with him to let her have at least a few pounds to feed the children, he beat her so savagely he broke her cheekbone and chipped four of her teeth.

'At that time he was also visiting the house next door, where he was conducting an affair with the occupant, a mother of six small children,' a psychiatrist said. 'It was a truly bizarre situation. His own wife and three children were starving and scared in one house, and next door were seven other human beings over whom he was beginning to exercise a tyrannical hold. There was no husband, he had taken off a year before Derek came on the scene, and the woman, Janice, was completely feckless and wide open to being manipulated. She was only twenty-nine, a pitiful sight really, and her helplessness brought out the worst in Derek. He used to torture her, tying her to chairs and tables, whipping her with a leather dog lead – he caused her all manner of hurt and humiliation. The children didn't escape his attention, either. He would tease them and make them cry, then beat them for crying. The oldest child, a twelve-year-old girl born while Janice was a teenage waitress in Cardiff, was a focus for regular torture, and Derek frequently involved her in various depraved sexual acts.'

'What shakes me,' said a police officer, 'is that nobody complained. From 1984 onwards, Derek Lewis carried on a protracted orgy of sadism against two adult women and nine children, yet not a word of it came to police ears until that unfortunate young woman was thrown out of her bedroom window.'

With no positive resistance Derek immersed himself in depravity. For four years he regularly beat his own children and the six next door. On one occasion the twelve-year-old's wrist was broken and she went to the local hospital, where they realigned the bones and put the arm in a plaster cast. When she got home Derek was there. He lifted her clean off the floor by her hair and demanded to know what she had told the people at the hospital about him. When he was satisfied that she had said nothing, he released her hair, grabbed the injured arm and tore off the plaster. He then beat the girl with the leather dog lead.

'It was the most sickening case of abuse I ever got involved in,' said a senior female police officer. 'Those children will never fit comfortably into the real world, they spent too much formative time in a nightmare. The boys were hung on doors and beaten. When we got them out of there they were covered in bruises and had deformed and broken teeth. The sexual abuse and the beatings went on for so long the children thought it happened everywhere. They thought it was *normal*.'

The charges against Derek Lewis included rape and indecent assault on four of the female children (one of them his own daughter), two charges of unnatural sex acts with his son, assault and actual bodily harm on his wife Eileen and attempted murder of Janice. Nineteen lesser charges were tabled and on his lawyer's advice Derek pleaded guilty.

'The court took very little notice of the psychiatric reports,' a forensic psychiatrist said. 'Derek was found to be suffering from Sadistic Personality Disorder, but frankly nobody gave a damn about that. I certainly didn't – it simply means there are ways of measuring the fact that he is a corrupt and wicked person. He's not mentally ill, the man is just a beast. One of the lawyers said he isn't fit to tread the same ground as decent human beings. The melodramatic tone aside, I agree with that.

'The judge put him in prison for fifteen years and I don't think that sentence was adequate. If we want to live in a

healthy society, we must face the fact that alongside
working hard to find cures and effective remedies for as
many ills as we can, we also have to lop off certain malignant elements for the general good of society.'

CASE THREE: *Disciplinarian*

Doug, a US Army drill sergeant, had a reputation for being
unusually vicious in his approach to training new recruits.
His aggression went beyond the customary verbal abuse
and extravagant threats; he devised punishments, usually in
the form of endurance tests, which pushed his victims to
the limits of their stamina and, in one or two cases, to the
boundaries of sanity. One young soldier, having been the
focus of a punishment campaign that had gone on for three
weeks, attacked Doug with a pick handle. Doug stood still
and took the battering, for which the soldier was punished
with six months in a military prison.

'Doug was a bastard to everybody,' another sergeant said.
'He was even a bastard to himself – I can remember one
day he put himself on report when he discovered he had a
shirt button open.'

Doug was a bachelor. He lived in off-camp accommodation, a small apartment in a quiet, fairly expensive
development where he found it easy to keep to himself. In
private he lived along lines as straight and unimaginative
as those he pursued when he was on duty. He was an
admirer of the Nazis, an apologist for Goebbels and
Himmler, and an avid collector of Third Reich memor-
abilia. His walls were hung with expensively framed repro-
ductions of late-thirties NSDAP campaign leaflets, SS
recruitment posters, Wehrmacht pennants and uniform
flashes. He had taught himself to speak German and had
memorised whole stretches of Hitler's speeches from tapes.

One day, he wrote in his diary which he had labelled 'Daily Thoughts', *the Nazis will be vindicated for what they tried to achieve in the thirties and forties. They did no more than apply a natural principle of civilised life. The strong have to manipulate the weak, it's a fundamental rule of life. The soft go under, they putrefy, we only have to look at nature to see the rule in action.*

On a wall in Doug's bedroom was a photograph of himself tied to a tree and sprouting arrows, like St Sebastian. The picture bore the stamp of a Münich photographer. The concept of punishment, given and received, fascinated him, and it was one of the few topics he could be drawn out on when he spent time in the sergeants' mess. Punishment, according to Doug, could have a two-way benefit, and when it was Doug who applied it, that was exactly what it was.

Early in 1991 he began to focus his corrective talent on a recruit called Edwards; a keen young man, eager to do well, but innately clumsy and slow to learn. This made him a natural target for Doug. In the first week of drilling Edwards was put on a daily punishment: he had to run three circuits of the drill square with a rifle held at arm's length above his head. In the second week his growing nervousness seemed to interfere with the learning process and made him clumsier still. Now Doug made him do four circuits of the drill square carrying the rifle straight above his head, as before.

On the third day of this gruelling regime a major sat in his car and watched Edwards as he pushed himself around the concrete square, gasping, his arms shaking, his legs threatening to give way as he entered the third circuit. The major decided this was an inhuman way to treat a recruit. He carpeted Doug.

'Recruits have to learn discipline and accurate responses to orders,' Doug told the major. 'Punishment makes them learn faster.'

That was so, the major agreed, but there were ways of punishing recruits which stopped well short of torture.

'Pain purifies,' Doug said. 'It's good for them.'

The major recalled how that had made the hairs on his neck stand up. He had Doug taken off training duties, pending a psychiatric report. Doug resisted, but in the end he had to see the psychiatrist. Throughout the interview he was uncommunicative and would only say, tautly, that if heads in that camp were to be examined in order of greatest need, his would be very near the end of the queue. The psychiatrist noted Doug's resistance to opening up, and issued an interim report suggesting that the subject might benefit from time spent on less stressful interactive duties.

The day the memo was passed to the major, Doug turned up on the drill square in combat gear, with a full back pack and carrying a rifle with bayonet fixed. He ordered the recruits at ease in defiance of the sergeant in charge, and walked straight up to Edwards, who was at the end of the front row.

'You'll never be a soldier if you don't take the burn,' Doug said. He then took a step back, levelled his rifle at waist height, and stuck the bayonet clean through Edwards' abdomen. As Edwards buckled Doug pulled out the bayonet and plunged it through him again, and then again. Edwards fell back with blood gushing from his abdomen. He died before the ambulance arrived.

Doug was declared sane by a forensic psychiatrist, but was diagnosed as suffering from Sadistic Personality Disorder. He was tried for murder and on the judge's recommendation he was sent to a special facility for the criminally insane. He is not likely ever to be released.

When sentence was passed on Doug he asked permission to address the court. He faced the jury and said it was soft men like the judge who were destroying the country. The day would come when Doug himself would stand in the forefront of those who would rescue the USA from the cancer of liberal thought and deed.

2
Pathological Jealousy

Sexual jealousy gives rise to hundreds of criminal cases handled by the courts every year, and it can be no surprise that one of the commonest recurring themes in psychiatric case histories is pathological jealousy. In an overwhelming majority of cases, the central feature is a persistent belief that a sexual partner is being unfaithful.

The strong emotions and unreasonable behaviour that are typical of jealousy do not in themselves add up to pathological jealousy. A man who catches his wife or girlfriend in bed with another man might fly into a rage and attack them, but he does that on realistic grounds, he has proof the woman is cheating on him. Jealousy is considered pathological when there is not enough evidence, or no evidence at all, and when the reasoning behind the jealousy does not stand up to examination. In 1955 researchers Todd and Dewhurst classified the pathological or morbid strain of jealousy, when it occurred in an established relationship, as the Othello Syndrome. Some psychiatrists still call it that; others use the term Conjugal Paranoia, but the official name, at present, is Pathological Jealousy.

Men are far more prone to the condition than women; one survey puts the ratio at nearly 4 to 1. A psychiatrist who has made a study of the underlying causes has noticed that extreme, unreasoning jealousy often nestles alongside other mental disorders.

'It likes company,' he said. 'There's quite often a connection with paranoid schizophrenia, depressive illness, alcoholism and drug dependency.' A number of authorities, he added, believe that jealousy in its pathological form affects as many as half of all patients suffering from neurosis and personality disorders.

'Apart from that, though, when there's no record of mental disorder, and when pathological jealousy suddenly puts in an appearance, it's important to take a hard look at the patient's personality. Pathologically jealous men often have a deeply embedded feeling that they're inadequate. They're forever evaluating themselves, surveying their shortcomings, comparing themselves unfavourably to other men. They see their ambitions on the one hand, their attainments on the other, and the discrepancies, even though they may be small, can weigh heavily. Men like that are highly vulnerable to anything touching on their sense of inadequacy.'

He added that Freud believed all jealousy, especially the delusional kind, was associated with unconscious homosexuality.

'But none of my own research or the surveys I've seen have been able to show any special connection between homosexuality and industrial-strength jealousy. One thing every practitioner will agree about, though, is that pathologically jealous people can be highly dangerous.'

One who was lethally dangerous was Terence John Iliffe,

whose case was cited in the 1975 Report of the Committee on Mentally Abnormal Offenders. Iliffe was committed to a hospital for the criminally insane after he had murdered his wife in a fit of jealousy. On his release from hospital he remarried, suffered a recurrence of his jealousy, and murdered his second wife.

CASE ONE: *New Man*

George Bailey fell into the same category of dangerousness as Terence John Iliffe, although George was in every sense a more complex character. A forty-seven-year-old hairdresser with a well-established and successful business, George became convinced over a period of months that his young wife was being unfaithful with a number of men. Over a period his jealousy became so inflammatory and psychologically destructive that it escalated into murderous violence, and the consequences were tragic.

Until mental disorder set in and began altering his personality, George had shown no signs of abnormal jealousy. To those who knew him socially he appeared to be something of a 'new man', keen to do nothing to cramp his wife's self-expression or restrict her freedom.

'He even encouraged me to dance with other men at parties,' his wife Lorraine told the police. 'He never liked dancing much himself, he was more the kind who just has a drink and a chat at parties, but he had nothing against me enjoying myself. I'd say that for the first two years we were married, George was near enough the ideal husband.'

During one of several interviews with psychiatrists, George explained how he first became suspicious of his wife's behaviour. It is important to remember that George never stopped believing that his jealousy was rooted in solid facts.

'She started to look different,' he said. 'She dressed that little bit more smartly, and her clothes were more provocative – shorter skirts, lower-cut tops, that kind of thing. She began wearing stockings and suspenders, too, where before it had always been tights. I asked her why she'd made the switch, and she said it was because she'd read somewhere that tights were unhealthy and caused cystitis.'

There were many other signs, George said, things only someone close to her would have noticed. He detected something in her eyes, a way of looking, difficult to define but nevertheless unmistakable, a mirroring of illicit thoughts.

'It was a distant sort of look, and her mouth moved in a certain way when her eyes went like that – sort of soft and glazed, that's how I thought of it. She got the look at odd times, I'd see it when we were in the pub, maybe, or out in the car together. It was never there when I knew her in the early days, or when we were first married. It was like she was thinking about something so hard it completely took her over for a while. When I'd noticed it a few times I started watching her, trying to work out what it was all about.'

Three psychiatrists, appointed by the court to determine George's sanity, could not agree on the underlying cause of his jealousy. One believed it was based in his reluctance to accept emotional responsibility. The other two were convinced it was the result of an overwhelming loss of self-esteem, induced by his wife's discovery that he habitually masturbated.

'I saw him at it a couple of times,' she said, 'through in a little room off the kitchen that he calls his den. I caught on to it one night when I heard this rustling noise and looked through the space at the door jamb. He was gawping at a nudie magazine while he was doing it. I was pretty badly shocked, really. It wasn't the kind of thing I would have expected, him being a grown man and all, and us having a normal sex life.'

Lorraine had a broad notion of what was normal. In later interviews she revealed that during intercourse, George had regularly extracted details from her about her sexual experiences before she met him, and he had occasionally reached orgasm while she whispered her richly detailed, largely invented 'reminiscences'. Her reward for such candour, she added wryly, was that George came to regard her as sexually depraved.

'He told me I'd been a slut, but I'd most likely been born that way and couldn't help it, and besides he'd taken a vow to stand by me whatever might happen, and he would honour that.'

When she first discovered George's solo sexual activity Lorraine decided to say nothing about it. She tried putting it from her mind. Then one evening she came home early from visiting her sister and walked in on George. He was sitting on the settee, masturbating as he watched a pornographic video. There was no way she could pretend she hadn't seen him, and as he blustered at her for barging in on his privacy like that, she turned defensive. She told him it would be hard not to catch him playing with himself, since he was at it all the time. They argued and George eventually became contrite. He admitted that he did sometimes relieve his sexual tension when he was alone, and explained the habit as a measure to stop himself from overburdening her with his attentions, since he suffered, he said, from being desperately oversexed.

The dissenting psychiatrist did not believe this episode was a trigger for George's abnormal jealousy and said that, on the contrary, it was a minor trauma.

'The most it could have been was a small factor contributing to his pathological jealousy,' he said. 'At the time of the incident he was already suffering from a sense of inadequacy. Look at the picture. He was a homely-looking man of forty-seven who had married an attractive, outgoing thirty-four-year-old woman. Following the glow of the early days when he was hardly able to believe his luck, a chillier reality set in. He became aware that Lorraine wasn't exactly in thrall of his thrusting maleness or his dazzling personality. It was apparent that his money and his large comfortable house had contributed more than a little to the fact that this blonde beauty now shared his home and his bed.'

Another difficulty surfaced. George had never before had a long-term relationship with a young, healthy woman. He had underestimated the physical demands of such an arrangement.

'He had to admit that regular lovemaking with her was a lot more taxing than he had expected. Marital sex rapidly took on the proportions of a chore. George was aware that he was not always able to satisfy Lorraine, or even to gauge exactly what she wanted of him in bed.

'To put it bluntly, masturbation was the kind of sex George was accustomed to, and now he turned to it more and more as a solace. Being caught in the act was a shock, but it didn't bring on any syndromes or do any lasting harm. It certainly didn't stop him. This practice was, after all, his deepest source of consolation.'

During a prolonged session with another psychiatrist, George admitted that although he had always been strongly attracted to women, on balance he preferred solo gratification. He argued that masturbation put him in control of the sex act, with no one to please but himself.

'Responsibility was clearly one of George's problems,' the dissenting psychiatrist said. 'He could exercise it comfortably in his business, but where responsibility involved the emotions or, in particular, the sexual side of a relationship, he was very uneasy. He would rather not be saddled with the need to fulfil his duties or to be accountable.'

George identified his reluctance to shoulder emotional responsibilities as a weakness. 'Rather than tackle it,' the psychiatrist said, 'he convinced himself it was something he couldn't help. He saw himself as a hapless victim of a weakness. So when other men came along with their superior capacity for affection and for sex, George reasoned that his weak and fundamentally immoral wife could not resist. That was an equation that made perfect sense to him, and his capacity for giving flight to his ideas made him suspect, and then swiftly believe, that his wife was unfaithful.'

He could find no evidence, but his certainty was immune to reason. At his busy salon he hired an extra assistant so he could be free at odd times of day to leave and spy on Lorraine.

'I had to work it out carefully,' George explained. 'Shadowing somebody isn't as easy as they make it look in the films. I hired a car, completely different make and colour to my own, so I could drive around the places Lorraine went without being spotted. Through the trade I got myself a good wig, and I wore glasses with thick horn rims. My clothes were all different, too – I kept a complete wardrobe in my locker at the salon. I reckon when I was fully done up with the clothes, the wig and the specs, I could have walked right past Lorraine and she wouldn't have caught on it was me.'

George belonged to the school of husbands who believe that their wives should not have jobs. During an interview he said he believed women with time on their hands were more likely to get up to mischief; the risk was worthwhile, nevertheless, compared to the damage done to them when they tried to tackle independence and authority, which were alien to their nature. However, because Lorraine complained that she had a lot of free time and too few ways to fill it, George had agreed to her taking a part-time unpaid job at a local day-centre for the elderly. It was here, George believed, that she first began to cheat on him. He had been tracking her to and from the shops and the day-centre for a couple of weeks before his 'breakthrough' happened.

'I always knew if there was something to find out, then I *would* find it out,' he said. 'If you persist in a thing, really stick at it and don't accept even the idea of failing, then you'll prevail. My Dad taught me that and I've proved it over and over again. I persisted with following Lorraine, I kept an eye on her every chance I got, because I knew she was up to something.'

He was hovering in the foyer of the day-centre, pretending to study the public notice board, when he saw his wife ten yards away, standing by a group of old people, deep in conversation with a handsome young man. As George watched he noticed they laughed a lot, and at one point Lorraine playfully slapped the man's arm. George went back outside and waited in his hired car. Later he followed the man home from the centre and discovered, from a plate by the door, that he was a chiropodist. A few inquiries revealed that he visited the centre once every two weeks on a voluntary basis.

'It was obvious from the way they had talked,' George said, 'the head movements, the hand movements, the smiling and the easy intimacy of it, they were more than just acquaintances. The relationship explained that far-away look of hers, or part of it. I kept following her and the more I watched, the more I uncovered.'

Something was going on between Lorraine and the deputy manager at the building society office where she deposited money for George once a week. George was convinced of that. Again the man in question was young and good-looking, and there was too much smiling between the two, too much warm familiarity for the relationship to be simply casual or above board.

The 'discoveries' caused George a great deal of torment. He could not concentrate, he went about his ordinary business in a daze and several of his customers commented on how gloomy and distracted he had become. At home he had to fabricate a pleasant front to keep Lorraine from being suspicious.

Even though the strain of mounting jealousy left him drained at the end of the day he slept poorly. As he lay awake hour after hour, feelings of sad apprehension alternated with restless anger, and he was compelled over and again to indulge in the pain-pleasure game of imagining his wife engaged in outlandish sex with her lovers.

As time passed and George continued to spy on Lorraine, the number of her illicit contacts grew. There was a newsagent who always, or nearly always, whispered something in her ear when she bought the evening paper; a security guard at the door of a bank appeared to know her terribly well, and George was increasingly sure that a traffic warden, who always seemed to be on the High Street at the same time as Lorraine, was making unspoken contact with her through a system of 'meaningful' eye signals.

At the height of this harrowing daily round of furtive

pursuit, of waiting and watching and drawing heart-tearing conclusions, George contracted influenza and was forced to take to his bed. Following a delirious phase lasting two days and nights, he came back to comparative reality dehydrated, haggard and firmly decided (the process of reaching the decision was something he couldn't recall) to confront Lorraine with what he knew. But when he tried to tell her, he couldn't, and he suspected he was in some way protecting his own precious deceit: 'It was as if I had to hang on to all that, my spying and the things I was finding out, to set against what she had, her infidelity, her secret life . . .'

When he was well again he noticed a number of changes in himself. Some were physical: at the time the flu struck he had been steadily losing weight and the infection speeded the process, so now he was twelve pounds lighter than he had been ten days before; he scarcely recognised himself when he looked in the mirror.

'I looked ten years older, my eyes were sunken and my skin was this terrible grey-yellow colour. I had no appetite and I didn't feel I had the strength to do more than make it to the nearest chair. But at the centre of me was this tiny fire, hot and hurting but *alive*, the only place in me I could detect any life, and that was where my soreness and anger were churning together in flames. That's how it felt, like a fire burning right into the lining of the man I was, taunting me to do something to put it out or damp it down before it got bigger and finished me off.'

When he finally returned to work he went back to spying on Lorraine, too. Over a period of weeks he made a 'certainty list' of the three men he was sure his wife was associating with in secret. It was important to write out the list, short though it was. When it was finished George put a copy in the inside pockets of his three suit jackets and his two sports coats. The first man on the list was the chiropodist, number two was the assistant manager in the building society; the third was the traffic warden who passed complicated eye signals to Lorraine whenever they saw each other on the street.

At this time George's problems took an extra twist when obsessive-compulsive behaviour crept in. The Obsessive-Compulsive Disorder has its own chapter elsewhere in the book, but it is worthwhile taking a moment here to explain the concept briefly.

An *obsession* is an intrusive and recurring thought, or idea or emotion; it is wholly a mental event. A *compulsion*, on the other hand, is behavioural; it is a repetitive act performed to relieve fear or discomfort connected with an obsession. The compulsion is dictated by the subconscious against the patient's wishes; if it is denied, he or she suffers great uneasiness, or mounting fear.

George's obsessive-compulsive behaviour was coupled with Magical Thinking, which is a belief that thoughts or actions can bring about effects impossible under the normal laws of cause and effect. George began setting himself exercises in mental arithmetic, connecting them with the notion that a wrong answer meant his wife would have sex in his absence that day, whereas a correct answer meant she would not. He was aware of the absurdity of this behaviour, but he could not help himself, and a hefty mental calculation became crucial to his ability to get through a day.

As time passed he made the sums harder and harder. 'In a sense I was uncovering a hidden talent, or an under-used one,' he told one psychiatrist. 'I was really pretty good. I would write down a list of six or eight two-digit numbers,

memorise them by looking at the list only once, then add
up the numbers in my head. When I got an answer I would
double-check it, in my head of course, then I'd go to the
written list, add it up, and if the two answers coincided, I
had won. That meant I felt a lot better. I'd experience a
strong sense of relief, with no anxiety at all, and for hours
on end I would hardly think about Lorraine or what she
was getting up to.'

As George's talent for doing sums improved, the periods
of relief inevitably became shorter. He responded by
increasing individual numbers to three digits, and by putting
a minimum of ten into each sum. When that became relatively easy he went up to four-digit numbers, and increased
the number of sums to two, then three a day.

'It seemed I spent most of every day doing sums in my
head. I had a penalty system where if I got numbers wrong,
or added them up wrong, I would add one more really
crippling calculation to the day's quota. It was hell, but if
I didn't do it I felt terrible, it was much better to put myself
through the misery. The really bad thing that happened
was that I started feeling jealous again, wondering about
Lorraine, imagining what she might be doing, and all the
time I was adding in my head, cross-checking numbers,
sweating it out and not being able to give it up in case
something bloody awful happened.'

The effort involved began to destroy George's ability to
concentrate on his work or communicate rationally with
other people. Finally, half demented with the strain of
mental arithmetic and the pain of his jealousy, George
decided to kill his wife's lovers.

'The change in him at that point must have been extraordinary,' a psychiatrist said. 'His compulsive urge vanished.
He was a wreck, but he felt at peace with himself. He had

vowed to perform the ultimate irreversible act, the act of taking human life, and that had appeased his devils for the time being. All he had to do was plan the killings, and he felt he had plenty of time to do that, he felt no urgency.'

Even so, George decided that the sooner the ultimate 'act of cleansing' was performed, the better it would be for all concerned.

'The men would be out of their misery, or they would be spared any, whichever the case,' he said, explaining his attitude at the time of planning the murders. 'Lorraine was bound to have made them suffer, sooner or later, as much as I had suffered. Also, by killing them for their iniquity I would be personally cleansed – the fouling of my spirit and my personality by her adultery would be cancelled.'

The thought of being punished did not trouble him in the least.

'I knew I would have to pay the law's price for what I was going to do, but that was all right. I regarded being locked up in a peaceful prison cell as quite a bonus, after all I'd been through.'

Twenty-four hours after the decision was taken, George set out in a hired Range Rover, armed with a twelve-bore shotgun, a pressurised garden-spray bottle full of petrol, a new clothes-line and a box of kitchen matches.

At a few minutes after nine o'clock, as the chiropodist came out of his office to take in a bottle of milk from the step, George took aim from across the street. The chiropodist's right eye, cheekbone and ear were blown away by the first shotgun blast; as he fell backwards, his heels skidding in his blood, the second cartridge exploded and tore away the calf of his left leg. In the resulting confusion George got back into the Range Rover and drove away.

An hour later the traffic warden, working his normal

beat, looked up from his notebook and saw the Range Rover hurtling along the broad pavement towards him. He turned and ran. Less than five seconds later he was hit from behind and thrown into the air. He landed on the road with such force that his leg, breastbone and skull were fractured.

Leaving the pavement to join the stream of passing traffic, George misjudged his speed and collided with a taxi. His engine stalled. As he struggled to restart, a policeman and the driver of a security van pulled him out of the cab. He was arrested after a spirited struggle and formally charged. At the police station he calmly revealed that after dealing with the traffic warden his plan had been to go on to the building society, where he had intended to get the assistant manager into his office at gunpoint and tie him to his chair, then spray petrol over him and set him on fire.

Because of the psychiatrists' failure to agree on certain points, their evaluation of George's mental condition was inconclusive in places and evasive in others. However, they were agreed that his morbid jealousy and its offshoots had become so psychologically destructive that he had developed a serious paranoid personality disorder.

'In the end,' a detective on the case commented, 'it boiled down to whether or not the man was fit to plead. During the police questioning he displayed signs I'd seen before – usually from malingerers and fly-men trying to line themselves up for a shot at a plea of derangement or mental breakdown. That's the trouble with fake nutters and the real ones, they're pretty much alike.'

As the sessions of questioning grew longer, fatigue began to loosen George's remaining grip on reality, until even the more lucid stretches of testimony (usually first thing in the morning, following a sound sleep) were peppered with absurdities.

'I wasn't really planning to take life away from those men,' he told an officer who asked if he had suffered any pangs of conscience at the harm he had done. 'It wasn't my intention to do anything so negative as to *deprive* them, even though some might say they deserved any depriving that was in the offing.'

What he planned was a two-edged thing, he explained. He had to restore his self-esteem and his peace of mind at his victims' expense, that was true, but in doing that he could ensure they gained something, too.

'I was giving them death, which is eternity, which is unending peace, and God knows that's something we'd all like to have, isn't it?'

Six weeks after his arrest, on the same morning that the traffic warden was released from hospital, and two days before the chiropodist finally died of his injuries, George confessed to a prison officer in the remand centre that he was going to kill his wife. He had reached the decision after long and distressing consideration. The whole mess, the ruination of his career, the loss of his freedom – even the terrible injuries of his two victims, were all her fault. He would kill her and he would say appropriate prayers to ensure she did not go to lasting peace, but went instead to hell for all eternity.

When the prison officer asked George how he intended to dispose of his wife, since he was locked up and had no chance to get near her, George held up his hands with their backs towards the officer.

'My nails,' he said. The officer noted they were well cared for, and quite long. 'Nobody can stop it happening, you see,' George went on. 'As they've been growing I've willed her life into ten parts and each part depends on the existence of a single nail. Starting today I'm cutting them. One a day for ten days. She'll sicken, and then she'll die. It's justice, and nobody can stop it. If they tried, I'd just bite off the lot before anybody could stop me.'

Following a further assessment, the three psychiatrists issued a report which said, in essence, that George's personality disorder was probably irreversible, and that he was now almost completely detached from reality. He was declared unfit to plead, and was committed to an institution for the criminally insane.

CASE TWO: *No Joking Matter*

Trevor, a professional comedian, was troubled by an intrusive mental image of his wife having sexual intercourse with other men. Many years before going professional with the comedy act, Trevor had been a United Dairies milk roundsman, and he had learned for himself that a lot of the risqué jokes about milkmen and married women fell short of the truth. He was perfectly prepared to admit that he had several times accepted sex in lieu of payment for an outstanding milk bill, and even occasionally when no bill was outstanding at all. The idea of his own wife committing adultery, however, made him shake with anger.

At first he thought the images were a by-product of his heavy drinking. He made a firm effort to cut back, and over three weeks reduced his intake by fully a third. But the images persisted, and they began to stay with him longer. He imagined his wife having sex with his friends, his enemies, his agent, even the management of the various clubs where he worked. The images were so vivid and their after-effects so pervasive that he began avoiding people who featured in these unavoidable fantasies.

One evening he walked into a club and saw a man at the

bar laughing heartily with a friend. The same man had featured in a vivid sexual image with Trevor's wife that afternoon. Before he knew he was doing it, Trevor had yelled to attract the man's attention. Loudly, he warned him he would be laughing on the other side of his face if he didn't watch his step. He then calmed down at a speed which startled him, and managed (he believed) to assure the man at the bar that it was just a gag.

Trevor finally consulted a doctor, who told him he should get more sleep, and prescribed a course of a mild tranquilliser. Trevor dutifully started going home earlier on nights when he could, getting to bed before midnight on nights off, and taking the tablets regularly. His imagination, however, grew more disorderly. He began to believe his wife really was having random sexual liaisons and that he, with his powerful intuition, was being told the truth by his ever vigilant brain. Until then, he decided, he simply hadn't wanted to believe the truth.

He couldn't confront his wife with his suspicions, because when he looked at her he was simply unable to believe she would ever betray him. When she was out of his sight, on the other hand, he could believe anything. The pressure of his jealousy began to affect his work. At one club where he was usually well received, his mistiming and fluffing drew jeers from the audience. Another club committee cancelled his contract. He went back to the doctor and explained his predicament. With Trevor's permission the doctor tape-recorded the interview, with a view to raising the case with a counsellor on nervous disorders.

'I can't get it out of my head now,' Trevor said. 'I stand up there telling gags, or I lean on a bar pretending to have a nice easy bevvy, or I try to talk to my friends on the street or before a show, and all the time it's going round my head, *she's doing it with somebody else!* It's driving me crazy.'

At home, he admitted, he was doing things he regarded as despicable. He was waiting until his wife was asleep, then checking her handbag for telephone numbers, photographs, anything incriminating; he had even begun examining her discarded underwear in the laundry basket.

'And I know I'm getting on her nerves,' he said. 'I can't relax with her any more, and the ironical bit is, I can't cope with the sex side of things any more. I just get started, then I get this picture in my head, her and another man doing it, and they're grinning, and panting, and I go right off it, I can't compete, if you follow me. I know it's upsetting her, she can hardly bring herself to speak to me some mornings, but it's not something I wished on myself, God knows.'

When the doctor tentatively suggested a consultation with a psychiatrist, Trevor balked. He had nothing against psychiatrists, he said, but if he went to see one it would be tantamount to admitting he had a mental problem, and he would never do that. He asked about the counsellor in nervous disorders – couldn't he see him instead? The counsellor *was* a psychiatrist, the doctor said. In the end Trevor settled for a more powerful tranquilliser, and promised the doctor he would come back to see him if matters got any worse.

Four days later, as he hailed a taxi on a busy London street, he saw his wife emerge from a tube station across the road. His heart jolted. She was with a man. He waved the taxi away and followed his wife and her companion, almost getting himself run over as he walked straight into the traffic to cross the road.

As he hurried to keep up, afraid he would lose them, he tried to rationalise the situation: his wife was a busy estate agent, she often saw clients and left the office with them, it was her job . . .

But this was different, he thought grimly. Twice he had seen the man touch her shoulder, and as they stopped to cross a narrow street he actually put his arm around her waist for a moment. This was her lover, Trevor thought, and the blood rushed in his ears.

At the next intersection he caught up with them and spun his wife around. Her guilt, he believed in that moment, was written all over her face. Before he knew what he had done he had slapped her, and as the man tried to stop him he hit him, too, knocking him down and kicking him on the chest and face. Trevor's wife was screaming something at him, her nose was bleeding and he felt suddenly that the whole world was caving in on him. He began to cry.

The man with his wife had not been her lover. He was a colleague from an out-of-town office who had been making a courtesy visit and was taking Trevor's wife to join him and his wife for lunch at his hotel.

Trevor learned all that in an interview room in a police station. Crushed with remorse, he admitted everything he was charged with, waived the presence of a solicitor and acknowledged the warning that he would probably be summoned to answer a charge of assault. When he got home his wife had gone.

'Even then,' he told his doctor, 'I actually imagined she had run away with another man. For about an hour I believed that. I couldn't see the obvious, I couldn't see I'd been driving her nuts with my weird behaviour, or that I'd really put the tin hat on it when I ran up to her in the street and belted her one and stuck the boot into her oppo.'

His wife never returned, and eighteen months later she

divorced him. Trevor has had a few girlfriends since she left, but he has admitted that he can no longer sustain a relationship without feeling unreasonably jealous almost as soon as the affair has begun. He knows his behaviour is unreasonable, but knowing that does nothing to alter his jealousy. He told his doctor that one day soon, if matters didn't improve, he might give in and put himself in the care of a competent psychiatrist.

3
Münchausen's Syndrome

Münchausen's Syndrome was first described in the *Lancet* in 1951, and was given its name because the wandering behaviour and habitual lying of the patients resembled the fantastic exploits of Baron Karl Friedrich von Münchausen, an eighteenth-century adventurer. Also known as Factitious Disorder with Physical Symptoms, the syndrome is a form of malingering where patients mutilate themselves in order to appear ill. When the deception is discovered, it is not uncommon for the patient to leave one hospital and turn up, shortly afterwards, at another. These people have been described as hospital addicts.

'They have this talent to present symptoms so well that they get admitted to hospital straight away, which is precisely what they want,' said a consultant psychiatrist at a London hospital. 'They are terrific actors most of them, and they do all their homework. They are familiar with the diagnoses of a host of illnesses that need hospital admission or drug treatment. They can give histories that fool the most experienced doctors and nurses. When it comes to faking symptoms – well, believe me, with some of them it amounts to a gift. They give it the energy and commitment some people would be glad to put into their jobs, if they could.'

Among the deceptions used to outwit hospital medical staff are samples of urine deliberately contaminated with blood or faeces; anti-coagulant drugs taken in slight over-dose, so the patient bleeds readily from the nose, the gums and the bladder; insulin taken to create low blood-sugar; certain types of soap eaten shortly before attending the hospital to produce an alarming (but harmless) fluttering of the heart. Many patients with Münchausen's Syndrome are associated with the medical and nursing professions. They are very often failed medical students or student nurses.

'In about half of all reported cases,' said the psychiatrist, 'the patients will ask for treatment with specific drugs, usually analgesics. They often get very awkward if they're resisted; it helps to deflect attention from their role-playing. When a test comes back negative, for instance, they'll blame the doctor and bawl him out for being incompetent, they'll threaten lawsuits and generally behave abusively. And it's all an act, although we don't agree on the extent to which individual patients *know* they're acting. They may not be so calculating as people think, because they sometimes give evidence of alternative personalities. They seem to switch between two different persons with widely different behaviour and attitudes.'

Other psychiatrists believe that the 'two-personalities' manifestation is just another act, as clever as the others, designed to fool those doctors or nurses who see past the first rank of deceptions.

'They're a group of gifted fantasists, clear-headed and

calculating,' said a psychiatrist in Glasgow. 'There's definite evidence that their need to be in the patient role exists for reasons that are far from normal. They might have been ill as children and enjoyed extensive medical care, or they have a grudge against the medical profession, or they have a deep-running affection for doctors and need to be near them. Whatever the reasons, these characters get into hospitals regularly and they cynically play hell with the system to serve their own ends. I don't believe, personally, that as a group they can be classified as mentally ill. If I accepted that, I would have to start believing other con artists were fundamentally sick, too.'

Hospital staffs in Los Angeles know a lot about Münchausen's Syndrome, so the successful deceivers have to be very good indeed to get themselves hospitalised in that city.

'And they do,' an LA hospital surgeon said. 'This is the heartland of falsehood and deception, remember. We've had them come in here with acute abdominal symptoms – not just one person but several in the time I've been at this hospital – with the abdomen covered in operation scars, some of them quite recent. They can do that, they can convince a professional, experienced, top-smart surgical team that an exploratory operation is what's needed, in spite of the suspicious hatchwork already there on the belly. Then there's the haemorrhagic type, wheeled in at high speed, bleeding from the nose, the ears, the mouth, the vagina or the anus, and sometimes, believe me it's true, they're leaking blood that isn't even human.'

The same surgeon described patients with apparent neurological symptoms, such as faints, blinding headaches, fits and loss of sensation in the limbs.

'I know of two fake neurological cases,' he said, 'where the patients, one a man, one a woman, had actually received brain surgery because their complaints had been so convincing.'

A variant of Münchausen's Syndrome is Münchausen by Proxy, where a patient or other adult deliberately harms a child to simulate a medical condition, often resulting in the child undergoing risky hospital procedures. The most commonly fabricated symptoms are bleeding from various orifices, pain seizures, loss of muscular co-ordination, coma, rashes, sugar in the urine (glycosuria), and fever; these can be produced by a number of ingenious means, some of them highly dangerous. In a large group of investigated cases it was noticed that many of the mothers had received nursing training, and some had themselves been diagnosed as having Münchausen's Syndrome.

No cases of Münchausen by Proxy are described in this chapter. The subject has recently been given broad and detailed treatment elsewhere, following a jury accepting that it was a causative factor in a case of multiple murder.

The condition known as *Pseudologia Fantastica*, pathological lying, is a frequent feature of Münchausen's Syndrome. Patients have been known to give a richly detailed history of the symptoms of their trumped-up complaint, so finely worked and accurate that a positive diagnosis and drug treatment have resulted.

'The lying and the wandering are the real pathological undertow to this condition,' the London psychiatrist said. 'They lie and wander even when they don't have to. It's as if that's the price of entry, the guarantee of success.

'These are seriously depressed individuals in need of an identity, and actively seeking one,' he continued. 'They are wholly self-centred, distraught and deeply masochistic. They are not seeking a cure, they are after the care and attention that goes along with a cure in medical surroundings. From a psychiatric point of view, therapy offers some hope of easing their symptoms, though it's too early to say if the good effects are lasting.'

The psychiatrist in Glasgow, on the other hand, does not think psychiatry should associate itself with this condition, which he regards as spurious.

'It is *not* a psychiatric syndrome, not in my understanding of the word. A syndrome is a characteristic combination of symptoms of a disease. But what disease is this so-called Münchausen's? It fulfils none of the criteria for a physical or psychiatric ailment. It is a branch of criminal behaviour practised by resourceful malingerers. It is also news to me that psychiatric treatment is beneficial to them. There is no evidence I know of which suggests anything of the kind. My own firm opinion is that treatment should be administered exclusively through the law courts.'

CASE ONE: *No Cause for Suspicion*

Judith, twenty-two, a technical assistant in a public health laboratory, had been attending an outpatient clinic for some weeks with a skin condition that proved very difficult to treat.

'At first it looked like a very nasty infected eczema of her face and arms,' said the dermatologist who treated her. 'There was an exudate, there were crusts, and there was inflammation. All classic signs, so I treated her accordingly – topical steroids, some systemic penicillin and a potassium permanganate soak for good measure.'

Instead of improving, however, after a few weeks Judith's condition began to change.

'It was crazy, really, now I think about it with the clarity of hindsight,' the dermatologist went on. 'But at the time it was just hugely puzzling. Her eczema began to look much more like impetigo, and that was the kind of change that just doesn't happen. Not in the real world. I took swabs and a few pieces of tissue – I remembered later that she seemed annoyed I was doing that – and I sent them for a path lab analysis. We got a call from the lab next day telling us we had slipped up somewhere, the request slip for Judith's specimens had arrived, but there were no specimens. I suppose that should have made me suspicious, too, but in truth it didn't.'

Judith missed her next appointment, and when she showed up one month after the doctor had last seen her, the skin condition on her face and arms had practically healed. But now she had something new. Broad areas of skin on her feet, reaching from the heels along the outer sides of the feet to the small toes, had become deeply ulcerated. She could wear only loose slippers and even then she had to walk with the aid of sticks.

'It was such a shock to see these lesions,' the dermatologist said. 'They were what we would call trophic ulcers. Normally we'd expect to see them in diabetic patients, or in people with nerve weakness and disease in the extremities. They were just totally out of place on this healthy young woman.'

It was a nurse who suggested that Judith's condition might be diagnosed as *Dermatitis Artefacta*, a self-inflicted skin disease. The dermatologist had to admit that in the circumstances it was a diagnosis he should consider. But again Judith's skin specimens failed to arrive at the laboratory, and she stopped attending the clinic.

Less than a month after breaking off her visits to outpatients, Judith was admitted to a surgical ward at the same hospital, complaining of severe abdominal pain and passing blood in her urine. On manual examination her abdomen seemed unusually firm, and she cried out when she was touched. An emergency exploratory operation was scheduled. Judith was being prepared when, by sheer chance, the dermatology nurse who had been suspicious of her ulcers appeared in the ward. She recognised Judith and explained to the duty surgeon that the woman had been attending outpatients with a strange and suspicious pattern of skin complaints.

The surgeon was more alert to chicanery than the dermatologist had been. He took it on himself to search Judith's property, with witnesses present, and found a quantity of 5 mg Marevan tablets, containing warfarin, used as an anticoagulant to thin the blood.

Judith was confronted with the find, and with the suspicions from Dermatology Outpatients that she was a malingerer. The surgeon even suggested to her that she had tampered with the lab specimens while the dermatologist and his staff were otherwise occupied.

Judith flew into a rage, accusing the surgeon of trying to kill her with his accusations. She promised, at the top of her voice, that the negligence of the nursing staff would be reported along with the doctor's unethical behaviour in falsely accusing her and illegally searching her property.

Instead of buckling in the face of the hysterical onslaught the surgeon calmly informed Judith he was going to call the police. In a fury of indignation she jumped out of bed, spluttering that she would not stay there a minute longer and leave herself open to any more episodes of malpractice and character assassination. She discharged herself within ten minutes and was gone. Later she refused to enter into any further communication with the hospital, or with

a Health Service official who called at her home to take
a statement.

Approximately two months later Judith was again admitted
to hospital, this time in Blackpool, where she now worked
as a dental nurse. She had left her job at the health laboratory because of what was described as 'a conflict of personalities', when she found she could no longer work with
the other employees, who, she said, were continually criti-
cising her.

'She was examined in the emergency department,' a casualty surgeon said, 'and haemoptysis was noted – that's
coughing up blood – together with chest pains and tenderness across the abdomen. It was a kind of confusing clinical
picture – but the woman was in distress, we couldn't be
sure this wasn't a huge emergency. I palpated her abdomen
and found it uncommonly firm, so naturally I suspected an
abnormal mass that was somehow playing havoc with various systems at once. A consultant surgeon examined her
briefly and decided we should carry out an exploratory
operation.'

Following a laparotomy, at which nothing unusual was
found, Judith's recovery seemed slow. She was sluggish,
complained of pain and needed extra analgesics to give her
relief. One morning when a nurse came to change the
dressing on Judith's abdomen, she found that half the stitches had burst and part of the underlying tissue was poking
through. Judith was quickly prepared for theatre again.
After the damage was repaired her recovery seemed even
slower than before. She complained of vague aches in her
limbs and spasmodic flashes of pain in the abdomen.

'What she didn't know,' the ward sister explained, 'was
that her whole background was being investigated. The

consultant surgeon wasn't too sympathetic to Münchausen's types, not when genuine cases were backed up on waiting lists right through the hospital.'

Suspicion had begun when Judith was on the operating table the first time. Her abdomen was clear, but her stomach was definitely in an unusual state of firmness. The surgeon decided to pass a gastroscope to take a look. When he did, he discovered two things. The first was that she had been eating large quantities of wet cotton wool; the second was that Judith's throat, at a point near the root of her tongue, had been deliberately scratched to create temporary bleeding.

'The wet cotton wool tactic is an old one,' the sister said. 'Soldiers used it when they wanted to get away from the scene of action. It creates a weird abdominal mass that's very hard to put a name to. While you're trying, of course, the patient can be lying in bed, being looked after and fed and generally pampered, and in twelve hours or so, he or she will have lost the cotton wool through the usual pipeline and the big mystery never gets solved. It was just luck in this case that things happened the way they did and the surgeon brought up a sample from the stomach.'

As for the scratches in Judith's throat, the sister had seen that before, in one case induced by puncturing the back of the throat with pins, another time by swallowing broken sewing needles.

'The story from the other hospital soon surfaced,' the sister said. 'Judith was confronted with the total findings and she nearly hit the roof. She stood up on the bed, clutching at her stitches, calling the doctors and me bastards, warning us we were sliding down the road to litigation. She stomped out of the place against everybody's advice and we never saw her again. The police tried to contact her to make some kind of arrangement for her to have the stitches monitored and eventually removed, but she had vanished from Blackpool, and there was no forwarding address.'

Judith's story ended a month later. She was found dead in an armchair in a lodging house outside Lytham St Anne's. A post-mortem examination showed she had swallowed a quantity of digoxin tablets. Digoxin is the most widely used form of digitalis, a drug used to boost contraction of the muscles of the heart. It was believed she may have been trying to simulate a heart attack and had accidentally poisoned herself. Deliberate suicide was ruled out, since more than twenty other more powerful and purpose-suited drugs were found among her property.

CASE TWO: *A Lonely Woman*

A middle-aged widow, Dinah, developed a rash across her face and on the backs of her hands which flared periodically to such an extent that she had to be admitted to hospital for intensive anti-inflammatory treatment. Although the condition had never been satisfactorily diagnosed, the anti-inflammatory treatment always worked after a few days, and then Dinah was sent home.

'That rash of hers used to have us taking bets with each other,' her consultant dermatologist said. 'The houseman would think it was one thing, the registrar would think another, and I'd over-rule them by saying it was something else again. It didn't conform to the rules, you see. But it didn't look like a self-inflicted condition, either. There are ways of telling these things. Self-inflicted lesions tend to be too hard-edged, they're inclined to avoid the eyes, there's a parallel uniformity to their distribution, and when they're on the face and hands it's always the left side that's more heavily affected, unless the patient is left-handed, of course. Dinah showed no such signs. Her lesions were of a uniform density from place to place and they were not at all regularly distributed. All in all they looked like they had been innocently contracted.'

Again, it was the events of the past that brought about the discovery that this patient could be classified either as suffering from Münchausen's Syndrome, or as a malingerer, depending on the point of view. A district nurse called Emma, new to the area, was asked to look in on Dinah and change a couple of dressings that had been put on her hands in hospital. The nurse had only been in the house a few minutes when she recognised Dinah. She did not say anything, and Dinah did not appear to know her.

Later, Emma went to see the consultant dermatologist at the hospital and told him she had first seen Dinah about twelve years before, in a general hospital in a town twenty miles away.

'I was a second-year nurse at the time,' she said. 'Dinah had been admitted with a weeping eczema that wouldn't respond to the treatment she had been having in out-patients. It was very nasty. It covered both sides of her face, her arms and the backs of her hands.'

Exhaustive tests were carried out, and meantime the staff did all they could to make Dinah comfortable. Not everyone was kindly inclined towards her, however. A staff nurse on the ward confided in Emma that she believed the eczema was self-inflicted. 'I saw her in the bathroom, rubbing it with something, she shoved it in her nightie as soon as she saw me, but I know she *can* bear to touch those lesions, even though she says they're too painful, and I'll bet she put them there in the first place.'

The staff nurse took it on herself to research Dinah's

background, which she was able to do largely by noting Dinah's National Insurance number and quoting it importantly every time she introduced herself, on the telephone, as an executive medical officer of the National Health.

'That staffer had a neck of solid brass,' said Emma, 'but she got what she was after. Dinah had been a medical student until she was twenty-one, then she dropped out when she went off with a man much older than herself, a divorcee, a university lecturer, and married him. He had dropped out too, he had resigned his job at the university and was writing a book, something about the forests of England, financed by some national body or other.'

The records showed that Dinah and her husband lived in various parts of England and Wales until, five years after the marriage, Dinah's husband died of pneumonia following a short bout of influenza. Shortly after that, or so it seemed, Dinah's career as a hospital addict began.

'She had a long list of admissions, all in different parts of the country. Our guess was, she was just lonely. She was young but she didn't want another man in her life. She'd actually said that to one of the nurses on the ward, she told her that she had been a widow a long time, but she had never wanted anyone to take the place of her dead husband. We believed she wanted company, and she wanted to be fussed over. All the same, she had a kind of grisly way of going about it. The lesions she had were horrible.'

Emma said the staff nurse had hesitated before taking matters further, largely because she had become sorry for Dinah. But as the days passed it was hard to stay quiet, especially when Dinah manipulated nurses and ward maids with a show of pain every time she asked a small favour, which was every few minutes.

In the end the staff nurse spoke to the consultant dermatologist about what she discovered, without explaining how she had done it. The consultant took the news with equanimity, and admitted he was intrigued. Above any other consideration, he wanted to know how Dinah had produced the weeping eczema. The staff nurse had a plan for finding out.

'She had noticed there were strict seventy-two hour cyclic peaks of inflammation with the rash,' Emma said, 'so she believed Dinah must be doing whatever she did every three days. She suggested we just watch her, then as soon as there was another flare-up, we should take skin specimens.'

The plan was executed. One morning shortly after Dinah had been to the bathroom, her face and arms began to swell and the eczema shone with exuding fluid. The staff nurse, assisted by Emma, took scaly skin samples, and dabbed pads of gauze on especially wet areas, so that the whole eruption was represented on glass slides and pads of gauze.

There was a long silence from the lab, and when the consultant dermatologist called to ask if there was a problem he was told yes, there was: they were having trouble identifying a foreign material on the samples. It took nearly another week, then the senior pathology lab technician, in person, brought the test results to the ward.

'Daz and powdered pumice was the lab's verdict,' Emma said. 'Dinah was creating an allergic reaction by putting detergent directly on her skin, then escalating the damage by rubbing in the abrasive powder.'

Emma took a look in Dinah's sponge bag while she was asleep. There was a zippered pouch inside, filled with washing powder, and beside it another, full of powdered pumice. A small chamois leather, stained grey from the pumice, was tucked underneath.

'She was confronted with it. She blustered, denied everything, told us we would suffer for this, then she broke down and admitted the lot. She left the hospital the same day and I never saw her again, until that day twelve years later when I walked into her tidy little house and changed the dressings on her hands.'

The dermatologist, on learning all this, decided to take psychiatric advice, as dermatologists often do. In this instance, however, the psychiatrist was less than helpful: he suggested the dermatologist simply humour Dinah and carry on as if he hadn't found out about her little ploy.

'I couldn't do that,' the dermatologist said. 'Apart from the cost of treating the woman and keeping her in hospital at regular intervals, there was the terrible fact that she was doing herself physical harm. Maybe she didn't mind about that, but I did, I couldn't go on being a party to it, not now that I was a *knowing* party.'

He confronted Dinah with what he knew. She took it more calmly than he had expected. Before he left she told him, haltingly, that she had finally, that same week, abandoned a lifelong principle and joined a private medical scheme. A silence stood between them when she had said that. The implications were not lost on the doctor.

'I told her, gently enough, that I was glad I wouldn't be asked to get involved in anything that might arise from her decision, since I don't take private patients. She replied that even if I had done private work, she would never have caused either one of us the embarrassment of presenting herself for treatment anywhere near me.'

In discussing Dinah's case, the dermatologist said that although he understood very little about Münchausen's Syndrome, he believed the sufferers must become very attached to whatever it gave them, in spite of the underlying bleakness. Dinah, he thought, had probably come to a more ingenious way of accommodating the condition, in the end, than most sufferers ever did.

4
Obsessive-Compulsive Personality Disorder

Psychiatrists regularly encounter borderline cases where reasonable behaviour is distorted to a point where it could be classified as mental disorder; on the other hand it could be a passing aberration, with no underlying disorder at all. Margins are often very wide and occasionally they overlap. Nowhere is the borderline harder to detect than in the Obsessive-Compulsive Personality Disorder which, at its mildest, looks like nothing more serious than over-tidiness and fussy attention to detail.

Sufferers from this condition show outward signs of being preoccupied with rules, with orderliness and neatness and an apparent inward drive towards perfection. Such people, because of the restrictions they place on their own personalities and their behaviour, tend to appear humourless and stand-offish. Very often they are regarded as prudish – women sufferers are frequently labelled 'frigid'. They take great comfort from routine and are often capable of handling massive workloads, so long as the work is largely routine and does not involve many changes of procedure.

Internal signs of the disorder are obsessional thoughts and images, compulsive drives to perform certain acts, anxiety and depression. Some patients have reported depersonalisation – they feel estranged from themselves, or that they are not real.

Brief descriptions of the more important symptoms will help clarify the condition.

Obsessional thoughts are unpleasant, often obscene ideas and words and opinions that the patient recognises as coming from within himself, and which invade his mind against his will. Because the thoughts are unpleasant the patient tries to resist them.

Obsessional images are clearly imagined scenes, often violent (mutilations, wholesale murder) or distasteful (butchery of live animals, unnatural sexual practices).

Obsessional ruminations often occur, in which there is constant internal argument about the pros and cons of performing simple, ordinary actions.

Compulsive acts take many forms, but four are very common. One, checking rituals – e.g. checking repeatedly that a cooker has been turned off, or a back door locked. Two, cleaning rituals, such as repeated washing of the hands, or repetitive house cleaning. Three, counting rituals, which can be spoken out loud or performed in silence. The counting is done in a variety of special ways, and it is usually associated with doubting thoughts, making it necessary to check a total several times to be absolutely sure it is correct. Four, dressing rituals, which involve a person in laying out his clothes in a special way, or putting them on in a particular order. There are often doubting thoughts here, too, which lead the person to start all over again, perhaps adding penalties for doubting, or for getting the order wrong. In severe cases a patient may take hours to get dressed.

Anxiety is always present in an Obsessive-Compulsive Disorder. After performing certain rituals a patient's anxiety will diminish, while following certain others he will be more anxious than before.

Depression in some patients seems to exist because of the internal conflicts of their condition. Others have recurring waves of depression that seem to be independent of the disorder.

The Obsessive-Compulsive Personality Disorder is occasionally responsible for sufferers finding themselves in conflict with the law. The following are two typical cases.

CASE ONE: *A Stickler for Perfection*

Daniel, a fifty-year-old citizen of Chicago, was seen by a psychiatrist after he had allegedly caused his wife to commit an act of violence against a neighbour. The neighbour, in the course of an argument with Daniel's wife, had remarked that Daniel was a malingering good-for-nothing; the wife responded by hitting the neighbour on the arms and legs with a snow shovel, causing a number of wounds that later needed stitching. Shortly afterwards, Daniel's family decided he should seek therapy, because his condition was a constant source of tension, and as his oldest son remarked, 'Now it's responsible for Mom whacking the woman next door, who knows where it could lead?'

Daniel did not believe he had any disorder in particular,

and certainly nothing that needed the intervention of a psychiatrist.

'It's been my experience,' he told the psychiatrist, 'that people needing psychiatric help *look* as though they do. Now I would suggest to you that I may look a trifle rumpled and I could certainly use a haircut, but I don't look like a candidate for your couch, do I?'

The psychiatrist suggested Daniel might benefit from a couple of sessions, anyway. Everybody, after all, had problems, and talking with an outsider could often go some way to ironing them out.

Daniel thought about it, then admitted that he had not worked for several years because he was 'a stickler for perfection'. That, he would concede, was a little unusual and could certainly be classified as a problem.

'But not a psychiatric condition,' he added.

Although Daniel was reluctant at first to talk about himself in detail, the psychiatrist did manage to learn that he came from a settled middle-class family and, according to his own view, he had a very happy childhood with no particularly outstanding features. As far as he could remember, he had been an entirely normal boy.

His wife, who was interviewed separately, had known Daniel since childhood, and she said he was 'painstaking and very slow' even as a schoolboy. He graduated from university half a year later than his contemporaries, because he could not complete his written project work on time.

Daniel went from university straight into a law firm, where he worked as a consultant on special aspects of company law. For a while he worked satisfactorily, but gradually he began to have trouble getting to the office on time, because he now had to arrange his clothes in a certain way before he put them on. If he made mistakes or inadvertently missed out parts of the ritual he had to undress and start all over again.

At the office he began finding it difficult to complete case assessments. He had no trouble getting them started, but he reached a point of 'fine-detailing' with each one where he was frightened to take it further, in case he 'unbalanced the perfection'. Finishing a case report was a nightmare, he said. It involved rewrite after rewrite, plus a constant re-jigging of the presentational style and pace; he simply could not let a report out of his hands until it was perfect. It was fortunate that he was working for his uncle's firm and was never in danger, at that stage, of losing his job.

After he was married Daniel began to have difficulty paying the household bills on time. Even when his wife sat him down at the dining room table with the overdue bills in front of him and put a pen in his hand, he still had to read every bill carefully and make a note to look up the details in his records at a later time, to make sure they were not being wrongly charged. This could happen as many as three times, with the bills only getting paid when people called for their money, or if unpleasant pressure was applied in other ways.

'In his middle thirties Daniel developed what I call the motivational brake,' the psychiatrist said. 'He intended to get up each morning at a certain time – and he truly did intend to – but he would get up later. Always. And even though he was late for work and knew he was late for work, he would insist on going through the ritual of breakfast, which never varied in content and always took the same unhurried form. He would drink two glasses of apple juice, eat a grapefruit followed by a sliced orange, then a bowl of oatmeal, followed by toast and coffee. He would read the paper while he ate his breakfast.'

After that Daniel would have a bath, which never took less than half an hour, then the dressing ritual would take another forty minutes.

'It must have been bizarre to live around this man,' said the psychiatrist. 'Some days he wasn't ready to leave for work until nearly noon. When he did get to the office he was always of value, because in interpersonal matters he was astute and his contributions were always to the point. His major problem was that he could not finish his case reports without being put under a lot of pressure over a prolonged period of time.'

Daniel got slower and slower as time went by. His uncle eventually fired him. With his severance money and some of his savings Daniel opened a consultancy of his own, but lost it within a year when he was unable to complete more than a small percentage of the projects he took on. With no job and no source of income, he simply stayed at home.

Domestic life was, in his wife's words, 'a black farce'. She had to work to support them and their children as Daniel got slower and slower. She regularly intercepted bills that had to be paid before Daniel got hold of them and put them in one of his numerous 'pending' files. A letter could stay with him for six months before he would even open it; following that, any action necessary in response to the letter could take up to a year to get started.

'Throughout our interviews Daniel simply insisted he was hyper-methodical,' the psychiatrist said. 'He could see there were problems, huge ones, but none of them, in his view, was serious enough to merit him dropping his standards of thoroughness.'

At the time Daniel's wife lost control and attacked the neighbour, Daniel had settled into a routine that did not vary. He awoke at 7.00 a.m., but never got up until about midday. He then showered or bathed and got dressed, by which time it was roughly 1.30 p.m. He next prepared his unvarying breakfast (his only meal of the day) and ate it as he read the paper. By the time breakfast was over it was usually about 4.00 p.m. He spent the remainder of the day reading law books and watching television. He would go to bed at 3.00 a.m.

The problem in reaching a satisfactory diagnosis with Daniel was that he did not admit to having many symptoms. The psychiatrist suspected there was a good deal of ritual behaviour beyond what had already been admitted, but Daniel said that wasn't so. He kept coming back to his conviction that he was nothing other than a man with a perfectionist and methodical slant to his nature.

'Psychotherapeutic treatment of someone like Daniel can be long and complicated,' said the psychiatrist. 'I wouldn't hold out much hope for improvement in that direction – and frankly I can't believe he would ever make it to group therapy sessions, even if we got him to agree to that approach.'

At the time of writing Daniel was receiving drug therapy with clonazepam (marketed as Rivotril in Britain and Klonopin in the United States), an anti-convulsant drug which is known to reduce symptoms in patients with indications of obsessive-compulsive problems. After eight weeks of the treatment Daniel's family had noticed a relaxing of his previously inflexible timetable, and his day-to-day mood seemed to have brightened.

CASE TWO: *Pressure*

George Berenson, fifty-three, was a transport manager with a major British manufacturing company. Over a three-year period George had watched the administrative workforce cut to a third of its previous size as the company 'rationalised and simplified' by a programme of staff redundancies.

'The pressure on him was terrible,' said a police officer. 'He was responsible for the smooth running of a transport fleet, the hiring, firing and conduct of twenty-odd lorry drivers, and a throughput of paperwork that had once kept two people busy full time. George's options were nil – he could either put up with the pressure, or get out and make way for a younger man.'

George's response was simply to keep on working. He went to bed early and got to work an hour before anyone else. He used the small time-gain to cope with the fact he was now doing the work of at least three people.

George's assistant was the first to notice his strange behaviour. 'He began walking round his desk once, a complete circuit, before he left the office,' the man said. 'I could see him through the glass partition. It was the same drill every time – he'd stand up, push back his chair, then go right round the desk then straight out the door. Sometimes if he thought he was being watched he would disguise what he was doing – stopping halfway round the desk, picking up papers and looking at them, then carrying on, stopping again . . .'

Other people began to notice oddities. One morning the cleaners saw George in his office, struggling to move his desk until it was directly opposite the window, which overlooked the staff car park. There was nothing unusual in that, except that George began spending much more time sitting at his desk staring down into the car park. His hyperactive approach to his workload appeared to slacken off, too. He would be seen muttering, shaking his head and occasionally getting up and banging on the window to remonstrate with other members of staff.

One morning when a driver was sitting opposite George at the desk, discussing a delivery schedule, he noticed that George kept looking behind him, at the window. From time to time he would stand up and stare down into the car park, shaking his head. The driver felt that George was giving him less than half his attention.

'And then right in the middle of me saying something,' the driver recalled, 'he yells out "Bastard!" then gets up and strides over to the window. He opened it and yelled down at somebody to straighten his car up between the lines. "That's what the bloody lines are there for!" he shouted, then he shut the window again and came back and sat down. By then he was pretty flushed, and his hands were shaking.'

Although George obviously continued trying hard to stay on top of his work, his preoccupation with the car park began to absorb the greater part of his time. It was now known among employees that if they left their cars even a little out of alignment with the guides painted on the ground in the car park, George would either shout at them from his office window, or he would seek them out where they worked and insist that they straighten up the offending vehicles. In spite of grumbles and complaints to other senior members of staff, nothing was done about George's odd behaviour until one morning the managing director parked his car with one front wheel completely over the white line. George stormed into the man's office and demanded he straighten up the car at once.

'I asked him to leave,' the managing director said. 'But he told me he wasn't budging until I went down and did something about the car. I'd heard he was behaving strangely, but I hadn't imagined it was anything like this.

He was white-faced, he was shaking, there was a blob of foamy spit at the corner of his mouth – the poor soul looked rabid. When I asked him again to leave, he leaned across the desk and grabbed me by the lapels. If I didn't straighten up that car, he said, he would march me down to the car park and make me do it. I tapped the emergency alarm with my foot and two security men came in and grabbed him. I got them to take him to a side office and I called our medical officer.'

George did not calm down, however, until the managing director went downstairs and straightened his car. When that was done, the change in George, according to the doctor supervising him, was like watching a man respond to a powerful sedative.

'He had behaved almost as if his life depended on that car being shifted,' the doctor said. 'When he looked through the window and saw it had been properly lined up, he went visibly limp. He sat in the corner with his head in his hands, taking deep breaths, sighing. He was embarrassed. He apologised to the managing director but insisted it was his job to see to the smooth running of the car park, among other things, and he had to insist that everyone, senior management included, complied with the regulations. That was as much explanation as he would make for his actions. Throughout it all, though, the most noticeable thing was his relief. That badly parked car had been like a huge weight on his mind.'

George was told to take time off and see his doctor. He responded huffily, saying he would make an appointment that day. He was back at work two days later. When the managing director called him in and asked what course of action his doctor had decided upon, George said he had been told he was suffering from an unusual strain of influenza, but it was clearing up now.

For a few days it certainly seemed that George's obsession with the tidiness of the car park had gone away, although his assistant noticed that he still walked right around his desk before he left the office, and he appeared to have developed a ritual with his sandwich box.

'He would take off the plastic lid,' his assistant said, 'and then he'd go to a lot of trouble to balance it on its edge beside the box. When he'd got it balanced, he took out the sandwiches, unwrapped them from the cling film, and ate them. The lid would stay balanced beside the box all this time. When he had finished eating he folded the cling film into a really tiny lump, dropped it in the box and put the lid back on.

'That wouldn't have looked too strange, I suppose, except for the lid standing on its edge like that, but what made it weird was, if the lid fell over at any time while he was opening the sandwiches, he would re-wrap them, put them back in the box, put the lid back on and start again. And once, while he was actually eating his first sandwich, the lid fell over. He just dropped the sandwich he was eating on top of the other one, wrapped them in the cling film and dropped them in the rubbish bin. Then he closed the sandwich box and put it back in his briefcase. His lunch was over.'

Within a few days of alleging he had spoken to his family doctor, George's behaviour towards users of the car park was as bad as ever. It reached a farcical peak when he had three people at the same time lining up their cars while he ran from one to the other, crouching behind them to see how they were doing.

'Finally, he pushed one man too far,' a police officer said. 'This chap had been asked twice before to park his car straight, with an equal space of tarmac inside the white lines on either side. The third time he told George he was crazy. He turned to walk away and George responded by kicking the man's car. When the man tried to restrain him, George began kicking *him*, and punching him and calling him names. George eventually had to be pulled off the victim and we were called. He was arrested on an assault charge that eventually went down in the book as grievous bodily harm.'

A forensic psychiatrist interviewed George and noted that he displayed a number of identifying signs which would qualify him for a diagnosis of Obsessive-Compulsive Personality Disorder.

'He was plagued by perfectionism,' the psychiatrist said, 'and apparently it had often interfered with his ability to complete work, simply because it didn't come up to his own high standards. This was before the staff cutbacks which marked the beginnings of his obsessive behaviour over the car parking. Throughout his working life, it seems, he was preoccupied with details such as list-making, multi-level job planning, office file systems analysis, timetabling and so forth – and all of it to a level of refining and hairsplitting where the point of the exercise was usually lost.'

George's wife approached the psychiatrist independently and filled out the picture. Her husband, she believed, had been in need of help for thirty years. In her view he had always been over-conscientious, and his inflexibility in matters of household routine (strict mealtimes, washing-up rotas, television switch-off time, bed times) had driven their three children away from home much earlier than they would otherwise have left.

'I come from a background where we were taught that when you make your bed, you lie on it,' George's wife said. 'Otherwise I would have left him long ago. In his twenties George started adding all these rules to our life together, and as I got used to one set he'd bring in another, and I think he got trapped in it somewhere along the line, he couldn't stop, he just had to keep doing it, and doing more and more of it.'

In the midst of his rule-making and his preoccupation with efficiency, George could be curiously indecisive: while he drew up the rules and the rotation of flowerbed and vegetable planting in the garden, it was his wife and one of his sons who actually did the work, since George could never seem to get around to making a start.

Another feature which helped clinch the psychiatrist's diagnosis of Obsessive-Compulsive Personality Disorder was George's principles of conduct, amounting to extreme prudishness, in matters of sexual morality.

'He never allowed me or the children to make what he called coarse innuendoes. Sexual jokes, even the silly harmless kind, were not allowed. It's not that he's religious at all. He isn't. But it's as if he hates sex.'

The woman added, with some embarrassment, that she had not had sexual relations with her husband for more than twenty years.

In the presence of the psychiatrist George eventually accepted that he had a serious problem. He admitted that he had grown to feel all his obsessions and his rituals and his patterns of thought to be a cage around him, both a prison and a protection. When he realised his job was no longer as secure as it had been, and that he would have to tighten an already tight approach to his work, his obsessions and compulsions seemed to multiply by the day. The car park was a central symbol for him; he didn't know why, it just was. He had decided (or he had been told, he could not decide which was true) that he could only cling to his narrow ledge of security so long as the cars were parked in accordance with the painted lines. All his other rituals had to remain in place, but they could only have their beneficial effects if the car park was kept in shape.

The magistrates found George guilty of causing grievous bodily harm. On the recommendation of the forensic psychiatrist they deferred sentence on condition that George submit to treatment for his monumental psychological problems. He readily agreed.

A week after the court decision George received a letter telling him that he no longer had a job. His severance pay was small – it didn't have to be generous, since he was sacked on a misdemeanour – and a number of plans such as the forthcoming holiday had to be abandoned. At the local employment office George was told that at his age, and with his recent record of conduct, it was unlikely they would be able to find him a job in the near future.

During later psychotherapy it became clear that George was becoming depressed. After two days on a drug regime to combat his depression, he jumped off the roof of a hotel. He died from multiple injuries.

5
Bipolar Disorder

Until 1962, largely because of the pioneering work of the German psychiatrist Emil Kraeplin (1856–1926), mania and depression were treated as a single illness, because the course of both conditions was the same in all essentials. The combination was called Manic Depressive Psychosis, or simply Manic Depression. Then three other psychiatrists – Leonhard, Korff and Schulz – suggested a division into three groups: people who had only a depressive disorder (Unipolar Depression); people who suffered only mania (Unipolar Mania); and people with both a depressive disorder and mania (Bipolar). Recently the practice has been to drop the term Unipolar Mania and include all cases of mania with the bipolar group, because nearly all patients with mania eventually suffer from depression, too.

Depression is a state of dejection and often excessive melancholy. There is a sense of hopelessness and feelings of inadequacy, often with physical symptoms. Mania, the polar opposite of depression, is a combination of exultant high spirits and boundless energy, with accelerated mental and physical activity which are in direct contrast to the general sluggishness of depression.

Mania goes beyond mere jollity and abundant energy, however. Sufferers become uninhibited and erratic in their behaviour, which may be aggressive and antisocial. They speak rapidly and usually, for preference, on trivial matters; often their speech is full of rhymes and puns. They sometimes have an impressive increase of memory, though usually for unimportant matters. They are easily distracted. Grandiose delusions are not unusual and patients often feel they have great influence over events and absolute power over their own destiny. The sexual drive is increased and sexual advances are often made towards complete strangers. People suffering manic episodes have no insight at all into their condition.

Nowadays it is believed that mania has a biological cause. The shift from mania to depression is known to be connected with increased levels of calcium and phosphorous in the blood, and the same change is noticed when certain depressive patients shift towards agitation and excitement. Treatment with Lithium salts (trade names include Phasal and Priadel) often has a striking effect on the condition.

'The bipolar patient is like a one-person drama, a walking compendium of moods and types,' said a Los Angeles psychiatrist. 'I've dealt with them for years, and I am endlessly surprised, in spite of preparing myself. To me the bipolar patients are very special and if I had the years and the financial security to study them exclusively, I would do that. We still have a hell of a lot to learn about this disorder. What we know, so far, is only the tip of the *tip* of the iceberg.

'When they're in a depressive phase it can be either neurotic or psychotic. The cause of a neurotic phase can arise from within and have no connection with what's happening in the world around them – highly successful and financially secure people can suffer from despair as easily as the bum sleeping on the street, and it's believed that genetic factors play a large part in that kind of depression. Psychotic depression, on the other hand, is a reaction to events in the patient's life and circumstances, usually some kind of loss.'

Mania, he pointed out, is the rarest of major psychoses. It is more common among women.

'To see someone swing from depression to mania is to watch a genuine transformation. I've been present a few times when the change occurred and it's pure theatre, better than anything anybody could cook up in a play or a movie. They look different, they sound different, you have a hard time convincing yourself that this fireball is the droopy character who was mooning about in the corridor just that morning. The same is true for the reverse, when the manic phase gives way to depression – it's suddenly a case of who is this? Can I believe my eyes? Bipolar disorder puts a strain on family and friends, it is a condition with such extremes of power contained within it that, very often, a sufferer will do great harm, both to property and to other people.'

Bipolar disorders, in the main, have a worse outlook than depressive conditions. Approximately 7 per cent of Bipolar Disorder patients have no recurrence of their symptoms, 45 per cent have more than a single episode, and 40 per cent develop a chronic illness. Long-term follow-up has shown 15 per cent of Bipolar Disorder patients to be well, 45 per cent were well but had suffered several relapses, 30 per cent were having a partial remission, while 10 per cent were chronically ill. A third of all Bipolar Disorder patients have chronic symptoms and show clear signs of decline in their relations with other people, and in their general ability to cope with their lives.

CASE ONE: *Emilio the Strong Man*

Emilio, a twenty-five-year-old amateur weight-lifter and body-building champion from Sugunto, Eastern Spain, was noticed by his family and friends to be undergoing a change of personality. He had always been a modest man, sober in his approach to others and having a tendency to stay out of arguments. In particular, he never made excessive claims for his ability as a weight-lifter, and shrugged off successes as no more than luck. But now he had told his brothers, his father and everybody else who would listen that he was becoming unbelievably strong. He also confided to his mother that he had learned the secret of divine happiness, and that because of what he now knew, he would become a very important man in Spanish public life.

'There were times, too, when he fell silent for hours on end, and communicated with no one,' said a psychiatrist from Murcia, who spent three weeks evaluating Emilio's case. 'His older brother believed that at such times he was very anxious about something, and reported that his brother sometimes wept, though he tried to conceal the fact.'

One evening, after he had repeatedly lifted a weight almost twice as heavy as his previous record, he went home, sat down in a chair and told his father, gravely, that he believed somebody in the town was trying to kill him.

'It is someone who knows of my association with General Franco,' he added, perplexing his father even further, since he knew that at the time of Franco's death in 1975, Emilio was a ten-year-old urchin with only the vaguest idea of who the dictator had been.

'Later that same night,' the psychiatrist said, 'Emilio left the house and went to a local bar, where he gave a demonstration of what he called his "gargantuan strength". He picked up a full beer barrel and walked around the bar with it held above his head. He then lowered it almost to the floor, raised it again, lowered it, and raised it, finally putting it on a high ledge; it took the efforts of three men with a ladder to retrieve it. Sitting down to the applause of local people and tourists, Emilio turned to a young woman at the table – he had never met her before – and told her his penis was as hard as iron.'

He returned home in the early hours of the morning, having spent the night showing off his weight-lifting talents, running races through the streets with local youths (beating them every time) and drinking copious amounts of alcohol, mostly wine. He went to the bedroom he shared with two brothers, sat on the bed and began to sob. The brothers had already left the house to go to work but Emilio's father heard him and came in. 'They are going to get me,' Emilio told him through his tears. 'They will kill me, and all because I love Spain more dearly than they do.'

Emilio eventually lay down and slept. He did not wake up until evening, and when he did his father went out and brought the local priest, who sat with Emilio and encouraged him to talk over his problems – in particular, this imminent trouble with the unnamed people who were out to kill him. Emilio obliged. He gave the priest three names, and explained they were agents of the devil, so the priest himself should be wary of them. After about half an hour of only semi-coherent answers to the priest's questioning, Emilio said he was thirsty. The priest told him to stay where he was, he would fetch water. When he came back, Emilio was asleep again, and he slept right through to the following morning.

'For several days after that he appeared normal again,' the psychiatrist said, 'though he was agitated and irritable. When his father asked him again about his belief that people were out to do him harm, Emilio shrugged and said perhaps he was mistaken about that. The father believed his son was on the mend, and decided to leave well enough alone. But after a few more days Emilio was suddenly charging around again, saying he had decided to run the length of the Costa del Sol for charity, and he wanted his father to organise local sponsorship for the shoes and other running gear he would need. His father tried to protest, but Emilio was too busy running about the town – wearing only an athletic support – to listen to the old man.'

Following an hour in the bar replenishing his vital fluids, as Emilio put it, he returned to his training on the streets. This time he decided that it was too hot to be encumbered by clothing, so he discarded the athletic support. He was arrested shortly afterwards as he ran stark naked past the church.

The police took him to the psychiatric wing of a local hospital, where an intern saw him and issued twenty capsules of a mild tranquilliser. Emilio, who was now depressed again, began screaming and throwing the capsules at the doctor, telling him he knew what he was up to, he knew when the agents of the devil were out to destroy him. He was forcibly restrained from hitting the doctor and was carried to a ward, where he was given a sedative injection. Again, he slept for many hours and woke up in a seemingly normal state of mind, though he was clearly confused about how he came to be in a hospital bed.

'He was discharged after a doctor had examined him,'

the psychiatrist said, 'and he went home thinking that he had simply been taken ill in a bar and had been given appropriate treatment at the hospital. When he got to his house, however, his mother attacked him physically, hitting him with a broom, cursing him for making the family a laughing stock all over the town. Emilio was bewildered. He took the beating without flinching or defending himself in any way. But when his mother dropped the broom and walked away from him, he picked it up and broke it into several pieces. He then stamped out of the house, went to the bar, and got drunk. At sunset he stepped out on to the main street with his arms held out wide, shouted for attention, and told the populace that he was going to demonstrate he was the strongest man in the world by lifting the donkey of the old Basque, Endika, and carrying it all the way around town on his shoulders.'

The attempt ended in a brawl. The donkey kicked Emilio when he tried to pick it up, and the owner, Endika, got his gun when he saw what was happening and threatened to blow Emilio's head off. A group of people tried to restrain Emilio while another grabbed the old man and disarmed him. Emilio suddenly decided they were all his enemies, climbed to the roof of a public building and threatened to jump on the main street and break it, unless they apologised for thwarting his attempt to pick up the donkey.

Emilio's father was brought to try and talk sense to his son, but when Emilio saw him he howled that even his own father was betraying him now, and with that he jumped off the roof. He landed on his backside and although a number of people laughed, and Emilio heightened the comic effect by picking himself up and stiffly walking home, he had in fact ruptured his spleen in the fall and was rushed to hospital at Murcia an hour later.

'I saw him here in our surgical unit four days after his

operation,' the psychiatrist said. 'He was lucky to be alive, and he knew it. He had been told by the nurse in charge that his cumulative behaviour had resulted in a dossier being prepared by the police, on the strength of which a committal order was being sought. He did not understand that, so I explained that they were trying to have him put away in a psychiatric institution. The news seemed to confirm something for him. He asked me if we could talk at greater length. I said it could be arranged, then he told me that it would please him if, after we talked, I could give him absolution.'

During the next two weeks the psychiatrist had to determine if Emilio was suffering from a schizophreniform disorder, or if Bipolar Disorder with Psychotic Features would be a more accurate diagnosis. To be schizophreniform, the mood disorder would have needed to be brief in relation to the other features of the illness; that was not the case, for Emilio's disordered mood persisted throughout his disturbance. It appeared that on balance, the manic phases had lasted longer than the bouts of depression, so the final diagnosis as it appeared on Emilio's record was Bipolar Disorder, Manic, with Mood-Congruent Psychotic Features.

Following hospital treatment with anti-manic medication, Emilio showed a return to near normal. Six months after his release from hospital his family, friends and the local police at Sugunto declared he was his old modest and unassuming self again. A year after treatment there was no reported relapse.

CASE TWO: *Off the Rails*
Karen, a thirty-eight-year-old divorcee, was taken to a private hospital near Cheltenham in Gloucestershire, England,

after she tried to kill herself by sitting in her car in the garage with the engine running, and a hose pipe leading from the exhaust pipe in through the partly open window. She was only saved when her daughter, upstairs in the house with her nanny, complained that the car was 'still running in its house' and she was afraid it would catch fire.

Karen had no concrete explanation for trying to take her life. She had a comfortable home, there were no money problems and her social circle was wide and varied. Part of the way into questioning her, the psychiatrist was handed a copy of her notes from a hospital in Brighton, where two years before Karen had been treated after trying to kill herself with an overdose of tablets. Confronted with this, Karen admitted that the attempt in the garage had in fact been her fourth.

'The first time I tried was after my marriage broke up,' she told the psychiatrist. 'After that, well, nothing I could point to, really. Just general fed-upness. I didn't have the energy for anything, I couldn't look after my own child. I get this despair, I sink into it, it's like glue, and I don't want to live, the very business of living, even motionless living, is too much to bear at times like that. Happiness becomes something I can't imagine.'

Over the years Karen had been treated with various antidepressant drugs, and she believed they had occasionally helped. Then she revealed that there were times, usually at the end of depressive episodes, when she didn't need any drugs at all to brighten her.

'Quite the opposite,' she said. 'I get so deliriously happy for a while I can't imagine it was me that wanted to end it all.'

During these 'up phases' as she called them, she would sleep no more than four or five hours a night, whereas when she was depressed she would never stay in bed less than twelve hours, and often as many as fourteen or fifteen.

'And when I'm up, I actually clean the house, I tidy the garden, and I telephone friends and organise all sorts of trips and events for myself and my little girl. I'm another woman completely.'

When she was pressed to recall how many of these high periods she had been through, Karen decided there had only been three, but they had been intensely memorable. She admitted that at those times she had always been careful to keep a couple of her close friends nearby, because she did not trust herself to behave entirely rationally. 'I always felt inclined to go off the sexual rails,' she explained.

Following the suicide attempt in the car, she was treated with the drug desipramine hydrochloride. After a few days her mood became elevated, then rapidly she appeared to become manic, talking endlessly, apparently unable to sit still, and being openly flirtatious towards a doctor and to a man cleaning the windows. No attempt was made to control this phase, it was merely monitored, with care being taken that no harm ensued from Karen's heightened mobility and excitement.

After careful investigative back-tracking on her various courses of medication, it was discovered that Karen's Bipolar Disorder was at least partly drug-energised; on the previous occasions when she had experienced her 'up phases' she had been on tricyclic drugs, of which desipramine is one. At other times she had been treated with other classes of drugs.

An attempt was made to keep track of Karen's progress, to see whether there would be any further manic phases with her continuing low-dose desipramine medication. Unfortunately from an investigative viewpoint – though fortunately for Karen's future – she met and married an airline pilot fourteen months after the suicide attempt. They set up home in Lucerne and no further psychiatric follow-up was possible.

CASE THREE: *The Merry Widow*
A sixty-eight-year-old woman was referred to a Brussels psychiatrist, as a result of pressure on the family doctor by the woman's son and daughter. Following the death of her husband the woman, Louisa, changed from being a retiring, old-for-her-age 'grouch', to an outgoing gregarious socialite who began throwing parties at her home and picking up the threads of friendships that had been abandoned twenty and thirty years before.

'The son and daughter didn't mind that,' the psychiatrist said, 'but they were worried that she was going seriously wrong in her head when they found out she was having sexual relations with a man in his twenties. She was also supporting this man financially, and he had told his cronies that he would probably marry Louisa before Christmas.'

At the first interview the woman was very angry that she should be submitted to this kind of examination, but by stages the psychiatrist won her trust and asked her if she could explain the surprising changes in herself in recent times. Louisa, who was wearing thick make-up, said she was now happy for possibly the first time in her life. As the psychiatrist tried to move the questioning to the link between the husband's death and the change of behaviour, Louisa kept interrupting, waving her hands as she spoke, and generally behaving with such agitation that the psychiatrist became silent and let her talk.

Louisa did not stop talking for thirty minutes. She described the amazing sex life she now had, she talked about the physical attributes of her lover compared to the paltry endowments of her late husband, and she told the psychiatrist that in all honesty, she was only now alive for the first time in her long life.

'She told me she only slept three hours a night, she went on endless shopping trips for clothes for herself and her young man, and she made love with him every day, sometimes twice, occasionally three times. She was experiencing orgasm every time, whereas in her entire married life she had climaxed maybe four times. She had even obtained a hand vibrator and used it when she felt sexually overwrought and her young man was not around.'

It was difficult to make any halfway scientific evaluation of the woman's state of mind, since she would not stay still long enough to listen to a series of questions, nor would she let the conversation be directed along lines she did not choose. The psychiatrist suggested they terminate the first session and meet again in a week's time. Louisa did not want to do that, but when the psychiatrist pointed out that it would stop her children nagging, she relented and promised to go back in seven days.

She kept her word, and to the psychiatrist's surprise she did not appear to have lost any of her verve or intensity.

'I had fully expected that she would have been on the down-curve of the manic phase,' the psychiatrist admitted, 'but she was just as bouncy and talkative as before, and she could hardly wait to tell me about her discovery of pornographic videos as an accessory to lovemaking. She told me she liked talking to me, it was like having a confessor without the pain of penance after the session. She went into detail about her young man again and revealed they planned to marry in November, a month from that date. When I broached the subject of her submitting to

6
Compulsive Rape

First the statistics. Most rapists are between 25 and 44 years of age; more than 50 per cent are white and have a tendency to select white women as their victims; 47 per cent are black and show a bias towards black victims, while the remaining 2 per cent represent all other races. Alcohol is a factor in 34 to 36 per cent of all rapes. American police statisticians have produced their own rudimentary character-composite of the typical rapist: he is a 20-year-old man from a low socio-economic group with previous convictions for robbery and other 'acquisitive' crimes.

The majority of rapes remain relatively secret crimes. Investigators estimate that on average 8 out of 10 rapes are never reported to the police. Under-reporting is attributed to extreme shame, and to the not-unreasonable belief that recourse through the legal system can often be as harrowing for the victim as the rape itself.

No female age group is exempt from rape. Recent records show a victim as young as 15 months and one as old as 86 years; women between 10 and 29 are in the highest risk category. Rape usually happens in the districts where the victims live, often in their own homes. The ratio of rapists who are strangers and those known to their victims is about equal; between 7 and 10 per cent of all rapes are committed by close relatives of the victim. More than 20 per cent of rapes involve two or more attackers.

Rape is an act of violence and although sex is the means of expressing the violence, the driving force is not always sexual. Long-term evaluations of investigated cases suggest there are three main categories of rapist:

1. Belligerent rapists (by far the majority), men who use rape as a displaced expression of extreme anger.
2. Exploitative predators, who attack impulsively and view women as objects of sexual gratification rather than as people.
3. Sexual sadists (rare), who are aroused by the pain they cause their victims.

A controversial fourth category involves rapists, particularly serial rapists, who suffer from an aberration of the sexual drive – known as a Paraphilia – where they are afflicted at irregular times of day and night by vivid sexual fantasies and intense, ungovernable sexual urges. The condition is called Paraphilic Coercive Disorder. Psychiatrists cannot agree whether it is a real mental disorder, or a justification for moral laxity and criminal behaviour on the part of certain weak individuals.

CASE ONE: *Dreamer*
A psychiatrist declared David Peters to be suffering from a Paraphilic Coercive Disorder when, at the age of thirty-four, he was arrested and charged with the rapes of eleven

women. David had already served thirteen years in prison on sexual assault charges. Between the ages of sixteen and thirty-eight he had officially raped twenty-six women, although privately he confessed to approximately twenty other cases where the victims had never reported the assaults.

Apart from the rape convictions, David had no other criminal record. He was a bachelor, owned his apartment and had a good work record as a packing-bay supervisor in a printing factory in Washington DC. He did not smoke, he drank only rarely and he had never abused drugs.

'He hadn't been so much as *suspected* of any other kind of criminal act,' said Dr Peter Lynch, a psychiatrist hired by the defence prior to the third trial. 'He was a model of sensitivity, a self-educated man of unusual intelligence and charm. It wasn't an act, I can spot a phoney at twenty feet and this guy was the real article. I also knew that I was not in any sense interviewing a criminal. He was a good man afflicted by a sickness powerful enough to take complete control of him for prolonged stretches of time.'

Throughout the pre-trial questioning David was completely cooperative. During interrogation by the police he made no effort to deny that he had committed the eleven rapes with which he was charged. His defence was that he was not in control of himself when the crimes took place, but was the victim of a pathological compulsion. He gave Dr Lynch and the forensic psychiatrists appointed by the court a clear and dispassionate account of his life up to that time, and shared his insights into his own varying states of mind during the twenty-two years when he had been raping women.

David grew up an only child in a disordered household in a lower middle-class area in the town of Alexandria, south-west of Washington. His father, a stock-controller in a business owned by his cousin, drank heavily and was frequently involved in bar-room brawls. He often beat his wife.

'He would hit her in circumstances where, in most other marriages, a man would just argue with his wife, or complain about something,' David told Dr Lynch. 'She would sometimes wait until he fell asleep, then she would get her own back and hit him with something. A couple of times she kept hitting him until he ran out of the house to get away from her.'

Once when David was nine years old, his mother hit her sleeping husband high on the bridge of the nose with an empty wine bottle. He simply twitched, made a rumbling sound in his throat, and slipped further down in his chair. Blood began to run from his nose down on to his shirt. The mother panicked and threw a jug of water in her husband's face, trying to revive him, but in the end it took a paramedic team to bring him round. He was taken to hospital suffering from severe concussion.

'That really scared her,' David recalled. 'She cried all that night, and for a long time after Dad came out of hospital she was like a different woman around him, and he was gentler with her, too. But after a while it was as bad as ever, they were drinking and swearing and hitting each other again.'

The couple were promiscuous. David's mother often had sexual intercourse in his presence with men who visited her in the afternoons. In spite of that, and in spite of the fact she was often so drunk she couldn't cook his meals, and sometimes went missing from home for days at a time, David did not think of his mother as a bad woman. He believed she was always good to him in her offhand way, and bore him genuine and lasting affection. His father, on the other hand, did not like David and often told him so. He regularly hit the boy and sodomised him on at least three occasions between the ages of four and five. David also remembered being forced to perform oral sex on his father.

In early adolescence David felt lonely and unloved. He had no real friends, since his parents were social lepers in the locality and other people's children were barred from even going near the Peters' house. Spending long periods alone, hearing his parents fighting downstairs, David would concoct fantasy scenarios of an ideal relationship between himself and a beautiful young woman, one who would be overwhelmed by him and live in thrall to his sheer charm and force of personality.

With the passing of time the fantasies became more erotic and they developed a repetitive, obsessional theme. David began imagining that instead of using his persuasive charm, he would force a beautiful woman into various sexual acts which she would eventually accept and enjoy; an important part of the scenario was a continuing warm relationship. David constructed six such fantasies (he called them his library), carefully detailed, graded to match different levels of mood. David could lose himself in these dreams and often – though not always – used them as masturbation fantasies.

'I knew the things I dreamed and schemed couldn't happen for me in real life,' he told Dr Lynch, 'not the way I imagined them. But that didn't stop me thinking beyond the drawing board, if you know what I mean. I started getting interested in the idea of actually doing those things instead of just picturing them and acting them out in my head. The urge got stronger the more I concentrated on the details, and after a while I guess it was an obsession.

I'd find I was thinking about sex all the time, for hours on end, thinking about doing it to some woman.'

David recalled dating only two girls throughout his teenage years. He went out with each of them only once, and both times he found the experience a strain.

'The rituals were so embarrassingly wooden. You know, going through the responses like I should, saying the right things, making a whole exhausting business out of just spending an evening with a girl I had no hope of having sex with, not for a long time anyway, and probably not even then, considering the old-fashioned kind I seemed to attract.'

The fantasies continued. As time passed they underwent alterations in detail and changes of emphasis. They became more vivid. Then the day came when David picked out a victim. At first he told himself he was simply memorising the woman's face and figure and the way she moved so he could put her directly into one of his fantasies; but part of him knew this was a move forward, one step towards taking the all-absorbing sex out of his head and making it reality.

'It was two days after my sixteenth birthday when I finally did it. I'd planned to do it on my birthday, but she wasn't where she usually was, she changed her schedule or something, and I had to hang on a couple of days. That only made me more excited.'

The victim was a woman of twenty-four, a hotel receptionist who filled most of the requirements of David's fantasy: she was slender and dark haired, with sensuous features and large brown eyes.

'Her looks were straight out of a comic-book story I read when I was twelve,' David explained. 'The loving wife of the hero was always waiting for him with a smile and open arms, and she had these Italian-looking features. I clipped frames out of that story and kept them a long time, and the woman, the type, became my ideal.'

David followed the woman from the hotel where she worked. As she took a shortcut across a parking lot to her apartment building, he went up behind her and put a hand over her mouth. With the other hand he brought a knife into view and told her that as long as she didn't struggle she would not be hurt. He then took her to a corner of the parking lot away from the sight of passers-by, and raped her. Afterwards, he assured her he had never planned to use the knife and that her life had never been in danger.

'After that first time, I told myself that was it, I wouldn't do it again,' he told Lynch. 'But it was like when I was younger and I'd promised myself I wouldn't jerk off again, the obsession came back, the tension built up.'

He committed a second rape three weeks after the first, in the town of Fredericksburg, and again he used a knife to coerce his victim. Although the threat of violence with a weapon was effective in gaining the woman's compliance, David swore he had no intention of harming her, even if she tried to resist him.

'What I told this woman was the same as I said to the first one, and it was the truth, I would never have used the knife to cause her any injury.'

The fact was that any sign of anguish or distress would have had an adverse effect on David's arousal. Pictures of women being tied up or forcibly subdued always aroused him, so long as he could imagine they were enjoying the experience. The least suspicion of fear or pain would cancel his sexual excitement.

'After the second rape, I told myself again I would quit. It was easy just after the event to feel like I meant it. As you would expect, the same old thing happened again. I would be working, thinking about not much in particular, and I'd get taken over by the obsession, all the sharp, clear images of forcing a woman to have sex with me, and then after a while I got the need that went along with the imagining.'

Two weeks after the second rape he committed the third. His victim was a young lawyer in Baltimore, and after David had run off she used her mobile telephone to give the police a description. It was accurate enough to get him caught as he climbed into his car by a shopping mall a mile from the park where the rape took place.

'It was creepy,' the rape victim later told a psychological counsellor. 'He gave me these directions, like we were doing a play or a movie or something. He kept talking all the time in a monotone, nearly a whisper, and when he was on top of me he said I had to *smile* at him. Smile, for Christ's sake. I wanted to scream, it was the only impulse I had, but he kept that knife on me, waving it back and forward . . .'

'David always wore a woollen mask when he attacked women,' Dr Lynch said, 'but his MO was more or less unvarying, so it didn't take the police computer long to finger him for all three rapes. And he didn't deny anything. A psychiatrist who interviewed him at that time tried to make a case for David having an Antisocial Personality Disorder. It was a simple-minded diagnosis, frankly, based on the premise that, in order to rape somebody, you *have* to be antisocial in the first place. The court wasn't interested. David got a five-year stretch – if he'd been older it would have been longer.'

David was released from prison after three years. His sexual fantasies were intact. His urge to rape, as far as he could tell, was also in place and undiminished by the threat of an even longer prison sentence if he was caught again. He rented a modest apartment, registered with his parole officer and successfully interviewed for a job washing cars at a gas station. On the sixth day after leaving prison he boarded a train to the Chesapeake Bay area. That same evening he raped a nurse in the ante-room of a private clinic and took the next train back to Washington.

David's orientation as a compulsive rapist was now firmly embedded. In the view of Dr Lynch, there was nothing David could have done to change that.

'This wasn't the kind of problem where a guy could muster his self-control and turn aside from his iniquity, as certain pompous airheads have suggested. David was being driven and he had no brakes. He was a cannonballing urge to rape. Conscience and restraint didn't have a look-in.'

David worked at varying his method of operation with each successive crime, and found this approach bought him time. He raped a further eleven women before he was arrested for the second time. By now he was twenty-one and facing the court without any useful psychiatric evaluation or even a reasonable defence going for him. His counsel spoke of David's preparedness to enter a rehabilitation scheme, but the prosecution's parading of raped women was much more persuasive. It proved disastrous to David's chances of leniency. He was sentenced to twelve-to-twenty years imprisonment.

Ten years later, in 1987, he was released on parole, bringing with him a document to say he had been an ideal prisoner with a flawless record of conduct, who could be recommended to any employer looking for a fastidious, diligent worker who took a pride in everything he turned his hand to.

'They also believed I had reformed,' David said. 'I learned inside that it was best to show a parole board a lot of remorse. "Learn to fake remorse," an old-timer told me, "and it'll cut years off your sentence." I think it did.'

David had no particular difficulty adjusting to the outside world, since it was a place to which he had never related on a realistic level. He simply re-established a live-eat-sleep environment, found a job to support himself, and continued with his fantasies. The difference between being in prison and being outside, he told Lynch, was that outside he knew he could have sex whenever he wanted.

A condition of David's parole was that he have weekly sessions with a state-appointed psychiatric counsellor, Dr Jane Harvey. They spent over 100 hours together during the next fourteen months, and Dr Harvey's observations and detailed notes ran to hundreds of pages. She had dealt with rapists before, she said, but none like David Peters.

'At first I couldn't find anything to hook a therapeutic line on,' she admitted. 'The man was practically a blueprint for normal. He threw up the kind of personality profile any mother would have wanted a son-in-law candidate to have. After five or six sessions I developed the feeling that if that single element were lifted out of his life, that urge to rape, he would be a model citizen. As things stood, I don't think I did anything for him. His condition was impregnable. When I talked to David I was only getting through to his head, I was nowhere close to communicating with the controls of his urges.'

Later, after David's third trial for multiple rape, Dr Lynch said much the same as Dr Harvey: David was like an ordinary man with a grotesque, alien attachment on his personality, and it could not be reasoned with or even reached.

'Nobody would deny David is an intelligent person, and his mind is more cultivated than the average,' he said. 'He's not a philistine, he has reasonably elevated taste in most things, given that he's spent a lot of time in the brutalising environs of the state correction facility. But all of that, his intelligence, his sensitivity, his grasp of aesthetic values, is a separate issue. It's a thing of the spirit, and if David was only a spirit, he would be a fine citizen. But he has appetites as well as a spirit, and his dominant need, as a non-spiritual human being, is to have enforced sex with women on a regular basis.'

Less than two years after being released from prison for the second time, David embarked on a series of sexual assaults on women which took him across four states. His new job, working as a courier for an electronics firm, meant he travelled extensively, delivering valuable customised electronic components too delicate to be sent through the mail. Because of the widespread pattern of his latest series of offences, it was months before the police – or, more accurately, their computers – began to recognise features of individual rapes that tied in with David's fundamental *modus operandi*. After committing eleven more rapes he was arrested again and went forward for trial as a potential three-time loser.

In preparing a defence case to show that David was the victim of a Paraphilic Coercive Disorder, Dr Lynch arranged that he should undergo special tests while he was in prison. One of these involved the use of a plethysmograph, a device for calculating fluctuations in the size of a part of the body, by measuring variations in the amounts of blood contained in the part. This particular machine had been adapted for penile measurements. It was attached to David as he looked at magazines and watched videos of women being bound and suppressed in various ways.

'He got erections from watching the bondage and domination stuff,' Dr Lynch said, 'but his arousal dropped if any of the women showed signs of pain or distress, or even plain discomfort.'

Tests on David's blood at this time indicated unusually high levels of testosterone, the principal male sex hormone. This tended to support Dr Lynch's claim that David was more of a victim than an aggressor, since he was compromised by his own chemistry.

'He admitted to me that his mind, at the times when he raped women, was in park. He was all impulse, all compulsive sexual drive. By then it had stopped bewildering him, but he was still mightily overawed by it.'

At the trial, much of Dr Lynch's testimony was undermined by a forensic psychiatrist appearing for the prosecution. He claimed there was no such condition as a Paraphilic Coercive Disorder.

'It has never been officially accepted as a valid diagnosis,' he said. 'The category is not recognised, it is a concoction devised to give weight to lax and wayward moral behaviour. In my view, which is shared by many of my colleagues, a man who dwells for hours on end on sexual thoughts, and then translates them into physical assaults on women, is simply a weak and fundamentally bad person. He is certainly not mentally ill.'

The jury went along with that. David was given eleven life sentences.

CASE TWO: *Secret Love*

Hans Grau, a twenty-eight-year-old roofing contractor from Bielefeld, West Germany, spent several days in July, 1982, watching the movements of a girl who worked as a kitchen assistant in a children's home run by nuns at Hillegossen. Grau had become obsessed with the girl after seeing her help nuns load a van with supplies at a local supermarket.

'She was my ideal,' he said later, 'an image of blonde perfection. I had dreamed about a girl like her for years, ever since I was a boy.'

Finally, on a Friday evening as the girl, sixteen-year-old Rowena Ditscher, left for home, Grau kidnapped her and took her to a house in the hills outside Bielefeld. The place was small and comfortably furnished, but as the girl soon discovered, it was as secure as a fortress. Every window was barred and both doors were secured with double locks and padlocked bolts on the outside.

'The house had been my grandfather's,' Grau told police officers. 'He died when I was twenty-four and left it to me, and for three years I dreamed of having my own ideal woman locked up in there. The house always represented that to me – a place where my secret love would be locked away.'

Grau told Rowena to make herself comfortable, because she was going to be there for a long time. On the first night he simply left her alone, after showing her around the house and explaining where everything was kept. The girl had been stunned for a time, unable to believe what had happened to her, but when Grau left she became hysterical. She tried for hours to break out of the house, but even the windows wouldn't break because they were made of armoured glass.

Grau reappeared the following evening. Rowena remembered that there was dry blood on his face, and the backs of his hands were scratched. He was shaking and appeared very nervous.

'He said hardly anything to me, he just sat in a chair and

looked at the floor. I asked him to let me go. He shook his head. I kept asking him, and eventually I was screaming at him. He jumped up suddenly, pushed me down on the floor and raped me.'

Grau left almost immediately afterwards. Next night he returned and this time Rowena tried to attack him with a kitchen knife, but he overpowered her. He asked her not to hate him like that. He told her he was really her friend. And then he raped her again.

Night after night he returned to the little house, sometimes bringing food, and on a few occasions arriving early with cleaning materials and a vacuum cleaner and cleaning the house while Rowena watched him, growing more bewildered at her predicament. Grau forced himself sexually on Rowena every night for a month. She said it was a long time before she stopped resisting, but even then she kept her mind separate, and tried to imagine that she truly only inhabited that mental space. In time, she said, her body became something detached as he used her, she scarcely regarded it as part of herself.

After three months, Rowena's family and the police moved reluctantly towards the conclusion that she was dead. Posters with her picture remained on billboards and in shop windows for more than a year, but finally they fell down, blew away or were removed, and the police stepped down the investigation until it was no more than a dormant open file.

'I thought of killing myself a lot of times,' Rowena said, 'but every time, it struck me that after I was dead there was no hope. Alive, I still had hope, even though it drifted away now and then.'

In the second year Grau's visits to the remote little house were more erratic, but he still visited at least three times a week, and Rowena grew accustomed to him, although she

never felt the slightest flicker of affection. Many times
she noticed that he would arrive looking dishevelled and
scratched; once he had a large bruise under his eye which
turned almost black during the time he was in the house.
Another time a clump of his hair was missing.

'He never talked about much,' she said. 'He came for
sex, always for that, and when I resisted he seemed to like
it more.'

Halfway through the second year of her imprisonment
Rowena discovered she was pregnant. She told Grau, and
he responded by bringing extra bedding for her, and asking
her if there was any special food she would need. Again,
in distress, she begged him to let her go, but he pretended
not to hear.

Throughout the pregnancy Grau continued to have sex
with Rowena, even when she complained of sickness and
the terrible discomfort. Towards the time when the child
was due Grau stayed at the house, leaving for only a couple
of hours at a time. He came back when Rowena was lying
on the bed delivering the child herself. He helped, tying off
the cord and cutting it, cleaning Rowena and changing the
bed linen. He then took the child out to the kitchen and
drowned it in the sink.

Rowena believed she went rather mad at that time. Her
recollection of events was poor, but she knew she had
fought with Grau and tried to revive her dead baby. In the
end he took the body away with him and did not return
for several days. Rowena had a fever and believed she
almost died. Her next clear recollection was of moving
around the house, humming to herself, and noticing in a
mirror that she had lost a great deal of weight. Grau began
to visit again, and again he forced her to have sex on
each occasion.

At the beginning of the third year Rowena began to

scrape away at the wood immediately beneath the casing
of the lock on the back door. It was part of her hope, she
explained, a small daily move in the direction of her idea
of salvation. The scraping was done with the dull point of
a table knife. As the months passed the groove under the
casing grew deep. At every visit Grau checked the house
for signs of escape attempts, but he never noticed the
groove under the lock.

'When the marvellous thing happened, I wasn't expecting
it,' Rowena said. 'I thought it would take a long time and
maybe do no good anyway. Scraping at the door had
become just something I did.'

It was the eighth month of her third year locked up in
the house. She went to the back door with her knife as
usual, and on the third or fourth stroke the blade suddenly
shot forward. She stood stock still, she remembered, unable
to understand. Then it dawned on her – she had cut clean
through the door. But the full glorious bonus didn't reveal
itself until she put a hand flat on the lock, bracing herself
to pull the knife out of the hole.

'The whole panel gave way. It just fell out on to the
gravel at the back. It made a huge hole in the door. I stood
staring at it, smelling the fresh air blowing through the gap.
I truly couldn't believe it. Then suddenly I did believe it. I
wriggled through the gap and started running. I didn't stop
until I saw people down on the road. I waved and they
waved back, and in less than an hour I was at the police
station.'

When Hans Grau was taken into custody he made a
lengthy statement, admitting that he had imprisoned
Rowena for nearly three years, and had murdered her child.
He also confessed to being the 'howling wolf' rapist, so-
called because he was alleged to have made a sound like a

wolf after committing each assault, although Grau dismissed that as stupid sensationalism. He confessed to thirty-three acts of rape over a six-year period. At his trial a forensic psychiatrist said he was a man who lived in the grip of sexual compulsions.

For the multiple rapes, the repeated rape and incarceration of Rowena Ditscher and the murder of her child, Grau was sentenced to prison for life, with no recommendation to parole.

After six weeks in prison he was attacked by three other prisoners, one of them a cousin of one of his rape victims. They partially castrated Grau with a hacksaw blade. Following his recovery he was transferred to a prison near Hannover, where he remains.

7
Post-Traumatic Psychosis

'A knock on the skull can do it,' a consultant neurologist said. 'Just picture it. You have a person who is a conventional, everyday, on-the-tracks member of society, who one morning slips on an icy pavement and bangs the back of his head. Now, if all his dark stars are in alignment, that's it. The change in him can be like no one ever imagined.'

Post-Traumatic Psychosis marks a crossover point between neurology and psychiatry. The study of causes is decidedly the domain of neurologists, who concede that much remains to be learned about the condition. Long-term effect and rehabilitation are the province of psychiatry, where the success rate is notably difficult to establish. Research programmes are continuously under way in Europe and the United States.

While cases of personality-change in the wake of a head injury are not rare, those where the accident victim turns into an emotional opposite of his former self are not so common. Even so, new cases are reported every year. The two which follow are typical.

CASE ONE: *Social Menace*

Dominic was twenty when he was involved in a road traffic accident near his home in the Dutch town of Leyden. A car travelling close behind his bicycle touched the rear wheel as Dominic made a right turn into a side street. The bicycle spun and Dominic was thrown into the path of another car. He rebounded off the bonnet and landed head-first in the gutter. On arrival at hospital he was found to have fractures to the right frontal and parietal bones of the skull, with bleeding from the right ear. His right femur was also broken.

Dominic was in a coma for twelve days, and he was kept in hospital for nine weeks. While he was in a coma his mother sat with him for several hours a day and talked about family matters as if he could hear her. During these sessions she often mentioned an ornate chandelier which Dominic's father was installing, with a great deal of difficulty, in the dining room at that time. Later, when Dominic was conscious, he kept using the word 'chandelier' in widely different and irrelevant contexts. He also used it in place of other words: a window shade became the chandelier, and so did the water jug by his bed. This curiosity of behaviour is known as Perseveration, a symptom of some schizophrenic disorders where the same word or phrase is repeated over and over, even though the stimulus that produced it has gone long ago. During the recovery period, Dominic was noticed to have other speech disturbances that hinted at the possibility of damage to his central or peripheral nervous system.

When Dominic went back home his parents reported a marked change in his personality. Before the accident he had been completely rational, notably even-tempered and a rather sober person for his age. People who had known him socially and at work described him as 'stodgy'. Now his mother said he was moody and bad-tempered, never less than irritable and forever arguing with her and his father at the least provocation. Sometimes, she said, he even manufactured the grounds for an argument.

'Worse than that,' a psychiatrist reported, 'he had become socially disinhibited. He would pick his nose and break wind in public as casually as if he were doing no more than clearing his throat. One time, waiting outside a supermarket for his mother, he felt too warm in the sunshine so he took off most of his clothes. If he was out and he needed to urinate, he would go to the nearest corner or shop doorway and just do it.

'And he remonstrated with everybody he met. He could not interact with another human being for more than five minutes without turning aggressive. He wasn't able to go back to his old job – he was a baker – because on three consecutive visits to see his workmates he had started arguments with them and had thrown a bowl of flour at the supervisor.'

After a particularly noisy scene with an old woman in the street (Dominic said she had bumped into him deliberately) he was arrested by a passing policeman and eventually charged with disorderly behaviour. He was brought before the magistrates, who ordered him to seek psychiatric help.

'He was very difficult with me at first,' the psychiatrist said. 'Uncommunicative, suspicious, insulting. But I stayed passive, I was careful not to give myself any combative coloration. Eventually, I think I represented so little of a barrier that Dominic saw me as someone purely receptive, an available and non-judgmental ear, and after a while he began to talk.

'It was mostly angry stuff, a lot of it disjointed and occasionally incoherent. He suffered from what we call 'knight's move thinking' – the knight is the one piece on the chess board that moves erratically. I put him on a course of Thorazine to slow down his chaotic thinking, and to see if we could effect some improvement in his general mood. But I suspect he wasn't taking the tablets the way they were prescribed.'

Dominic's behaviour deteriorated steadily in the following year. He gradually became secretive, keeping to his room and accusing his parents of prying whenever they asked him personal questions. He managed to keep up monthly visits to the psychiatrist, and at those sessions he began to express powerful hostility towards women, openly expressing malice towards his mother and a female cousin who visited their home.

'I think some bad sexual encounter had prompted that,' the psychiatrist said, 'although he denied any contact with women. In fact he denied any interest in sex at all, which could have been a side-effect of the tablets – I had switched him to haloperidol by then, but I didn't believe he was taking them any more regularly than he took the others. It is quite possible, of course, that he was just lying to me at that time.'

Dominic eventually managed to get a job working in the unpacking bay at a factory. All he had to do all day was cut open boxes and stack the contents on shelves. He did not have to speak to anyone. The work appeared to suit him. About a month after he got the job his father visited the psychiatrist. He reported that Dominic had been bringing home pornographic magazines, as many as a dozen a week. Also, although Dominic was extremely secretive at home and stayed in his room most of the time, his father knew he was masturbating excessively.

'This is a young man,' his father said plaintively, 'who made a virtue of treating his body and his mind with respect, until that accident.'

Eventually, Dominic was found masturbating in the open doorway of the unpacking bay at the factory. He was suspended from work. The psychiatrist arranged to have him admitted to a psychiatric rehabilitation unit. He discharged himself from there after a month.

'For six weeks after that his parents went through hell with him,' the psychiatrist said. 'He was disruptive, playing loud music at the dead of night, locking himself in the bathroom and flushing the toilet twenty or thirty times in succession, then filling the bath to the very top, so that when he flopped into it the water spilled on the floor and seeped through the sitting-room ceiling. He saved up his urine in bottles and then poured it on the lawn his father was so proud of, killing huge patches of grass. Many times he threatened his father with violence, and he ignored his mother completely. He lived on hamburgers, bags of corn snacks and soft drinks, and wouldn't eat the food his mother cooked for him.'

Dominic was eventually placed in a well-guarded psychiatric ward in a general hospital. While he was there he continued to be disruptive. He made sexual advances to the nurses and tried to rape a young medical student. He was moved to another ward where security was much tighter, and while he was there he underwent extensive neurological investigation. He was provisionally diagnosed as suffering from a frontal-lobe lesion of the brain, probably accountable to his accident.

'The frontal lobe is connected with the brain areas governing movement, emotions and the senses,' the neurologist explained. 'It is critical to personality, memory, judgement and other higher functions. Damage in that area can produce uninhibited behaviour, irritability and depression, among other deficits.'

One condition sometimes produced by frontal lobe damage is called *Witzelsucht*, where the subject indulges in feeble, inappropriate humour; Dominic certainly appeared to be suffering from that. In his communicative phases he regularly made puns that no one could understand, he told nurses lengthy jokes with apparently no punch-lines (even though they made Dominic laugh) and at the time of the Lockerbie disaster in Britain, when staff and several patients wept at the news on television, Dominic remarked that at least the American airports would not be so busy that night, and laughed uproariously.

A psychological assessment carried out shortly after the neurological tests showed that Dominic had average intellectual functioning, with some deficiencies of verbal and visual memory, and his fluency was considered poor. He continued to repeat fixed phrases and words.

'Most of the time he was still withdrawn,' said the psychiatrist, 'his social behaviour was *definitely* inadequate – he masturbated wherever and whenever he felt like it – and he had become increasingly preoccupied with sexual fantasies. He said he had a strong desire to commit buggery on young girls, and he believed he would enjoy observing their pain and embarrassment.'

Dominic was given the drug Depo Provera to suppress his sexual drive, and attempts were made to transfer him to a rehabilitation unit. However, during that time the haloperidol therapy, which had been regular since he went to the hospital, was reduced; his behaviour promptly became unstable. He started attacking nursing staff again.

A later attempt was made to rehabilitate him, but that was only partially successful. He still assaulted staff and other patients, and on several occasions he exposed himself to visitors to the unit.

When a restructuring of health amenities in the area finally closed the special ward where Dominic was being kept, he was transferred to a small and relatively secure psychiatric hospital, where he stayed for nearly five years. There were problems in the early stages but finally he settled in. However, whenever any reduction of his tranquilliser therapy was attempted, he always became unstable until it was restored. His grasp of reality, even in his relatively stable periods, was not good.

'He had delusions that he was being persecuted by the staff and other patients,' the psychiatrist said. 'He said they were trying to poison him, and he produced evidence, so-called swabs taken from food bowls and cups. He was hearing voices, too. One of them was God, he thought, or it could have been an Archangel. Whoever it was, this particular voice was telling Dominic he should kill certain notable politicians and major clergy, strictly for his own safety.'

During a period when his haloperidol medication was being reduced, Dominic leaned out of a window one morning and jerked a ladder a window-cleaner was working on. The man fell off and broke his shoulder. The police were called and during the subsequent investigation a forensic psychiatrist, Han Leowe, was asked to evaluate Dominic's level of sanity.

'He displayed psychotic symptoms all right,' Dr Leowe said, 'but frankly it was hard to say to what extent they were the after-effects of his brain injury, and how much was due to the symptoms he had picked up off other patients.'

Dr Leowe suspected that Dominic hid behind a facade of madness much bigger than his real problem.

'I also suspect – no, to be blunt, I *firmly believe* he was managing to fool his psychiatrist and the nursing staff at the unit. Maybe his reason for doing that was created by his accident, but I don't think he's anything like so badly damaged by the head injuries as he makes out. Let's say the accident turned him into a bad man, after he had been a distinctly good man. That is perfectly believable. He's undergone a change of personality that has made him a vicious, sex-obsessed lout, a dangerous one who should be kept away from society, because he doesn't like people one little bit. But that doesn't make him classifiable as mentally ill. Through sheer accident, he's become a nasty piece of work who can be suppressed by drugs, but when he's taken off the drugs he starts going antisocial again, as all bad men will.'

There was prolonged argument between Dr Leowe and Dominic's regular psychiatrist about just how far Dominic had been mentally disordered by his accident. It was the 'mad or bad' argument again. In Dr Leowe's view Dominic was intelligent, calculating and manipulative, and he clearly impersonated other patients' symptoms and patterns of behaviour – there was a good deal of evidence for that. The other psychiatrist believed brain injury had disordered Dominic's mental processes to the point where he had no sane responsibility for any of his actions.

Whatever the truth of the issue, Dominic continued to be a considerable danger to other people. When he was left without supervision he tried to assault women, or to commit some other outrage with a sexual and/or violent motive. He appeared to have two distinct states, and only two: in one, he was so suppressed by haloperidol and Depo

Provera that he was as good as inanimate, while in the other he was actively malignant and could not be left unsupervised for any length of time.

At Christmas 1992 Dominic cut his wrists on the edge of a broken drinking glass. Six weeks later, however, because he had been showing a remarkable improvement in his behaviour, he was allowed out on supervised leave. On a busy main street he tried to push the guard escorting him under the wheels of a taxi.

In June 1993 he was transferred to a hospital for the criminally insane. After six weeks there he fatally electrocuted himself by sticking a metal leg from a pair of sunglasses into a live wall socket.

CASE TWO: *A Short Fuse*

In 1967 a female police detective, Eva Kurtz, was ambushed by a burglar she had been trailing near the docks in Hamburg, Northwest Germany. He leapt on her as she climbed into the cabin of a crane and hit her three times on the side of the head with a short length of steel pipe. Eva's skull was eventually found to be fractured in three places. She lay undiscovered in the crane for six hours and when she was eventually rushed to hospital she had lost three pints of blood from a haemorrhage in one ear and seepage from her wounds.

In a statement to the press, doctors said it was Eva's youth – she was twenty-four at the time of the assault – and her general level of fitness that saved her life. However, although she was brought back to good physical health and eventually returned to duty with the Hamburg police, Eva had been permanently damaged by her injuries.

When surgeons performed an emergency operation to remove a huge blood clot pressing on her brain, they had noted a tearing injury to the temporal area of the cerebral cortex – the thin layer of grey matter covering the hemispheres of the brain. The degree of injury did not seem too severe, and it was agreed that it should be left to heal unaided, since interference in such a region could turn a minor injury into a fatal one. In a short time, this damage to the cortex was to play havoc with Eva's personality.

She had been back at work for only a few hours when colleagues began to notice changes in her behaviour. Her voice, once light and melodic, was now flat and monotonous; Eva did not seem to be aware of this.

'It was what we call Aprosody,' a forensic psychiatrist explained. 'It often happens when there's been injury to the temporal cortex. She had periodic lapses of memory, too, and a bunch of other reactions that clearly pointed to brain injury. The trouble is, she didn't start getting help until a lot of damage had been done.'

The main harm was done to Eva's reputation. On her first major arrest after going back to work, a prisoner tried to make a run for it as he was bundled into a police car; he was caught by a uniformed police officer before he got twenty feet away, but Eva's reaction to his act of resistance was to fly into a rage.

'She jumped on the prisoner and started pulling his hair,' a fellow officer recalled. 'She was screaming at him as she tried to make him bald, getting hold of big chunks of hair and telling him he was every kind of bastard and a lot of other things a lady shouldn't call anybody.'

Eva was pulled off the terrified prisoner and her rage subsided as fast as it had appeared. Later, while she was making out her report, she began to read her notes then sat back, looking startled. She beckoned another female officer and asked her to look at the notes.

'Can you read what's written there?' she asked.

The woman said she could, and she read it aloud. Eva took back the notebook and stared at it. Shaking her head, she left the office and got herself a cup of coffee from a machine in the corridor. When she came back she sat down and looked at the book again. Her superior officer, who had been watching what happened, asked her if everything was all right. She said yes, it was; for some reason, she hadn't been able to understand the words in her notes, but now they were perfectly clear.

The rage reaction showed itself again a few days later when Eva was questioning the female manager of a shop about a customer who had passed counterfeit banknotes. The woman gave a description of the man, Eva wrote it down and then a few minutes later, as was the usual practice, she asked for the description to be repeated – discrepancies of memory often show up at interview and it is sensible practice to pinpoint and eliminate them wherever possible. However, when the shop manager in this case said the man had worn a brown jacket, when earlier she had said it was maroon, Eva glared at her, then slapped her notebook down on the counter. A male colleague recalled what happened next.

'She demanded to know if the woman was deliberately trying to confuse and mislead the police,' he said. 'When the woman tried to say she was sorry Eva interrupted her and said she might as well confess there and then that she was trying to waste police time. It would go easier with her if she admitted it straight away, rather than dragging the matter out. The woman was in tears by then. That seemed to make Eva worse. She caught the woman by the shoulders and began shaking her. That's when I intervened. Eva looked at me as if she would gladly have shot me. But she backed off, and five minutes later she was behaving as if the whole thing had never happened.'

Eva's private life had undergone a few startling changes, too. She was single, with no serious male attachments, and shared a flat with her sister, who was a schoolteacher. Until the time of the attack which put her in hospital, Eva had operated to a tight sexual code: she did not sleep with a man unless she knew him very well, and while she was sleeping with one man she would not consider sleeping with another. Now, according to her sister, all of that had gone by the board.

'She actually picked up a man in a bar and brought him back to the flat. He was terrible, too, nothing like the kind she usually fancied. He was younger than her, a long-haired biker type, and whatever they were getting up to in her room, it sounded like it was causing him a lot of pain.'

At the end of her first month back at work Eva lost her temper again and this time the incident could not be overlooked. She was taking a statement from a prisoner, a young woman found in possession of a kilo of cannabis resin. She was very nervous as she gave her statement and kept fiddling with the ends of her long hair. She told Eva the cannabis had been left with her for safe-keeping by a boyfriend, and she hadn't know what it was; if she *had* known, she said, she would never have had anything to do with the stuff. The same male officer who had intervened before when Eva lost her temper was with her on this occasion, and he saw the trouble coming.

Eva sat staring when the girl had finished telling her story.

'Do you expect me to believe that?' she said.

The girl shrugged and went on fiddling with her hair. Eva watched her, then suddenly slapped the girl's hand away from her hair. The male officer made a move towards Eva and that seemed to precipitate a rush of events. The prisoner slapped Eva on the hand, a small, half-hearted retaliation; Eva stood up and swung her bunched fist in an arc, hitting the girl on the cheek. She did it again, hitting her mouth this time and cracking a tooth. When the girl stood up to get out of Eva's way the male officer caught Eva round the waist from behind. She lashed out with her feet and kicked the prisoner savagely in the stomach. Then she went limp in the officer's arms, and when he got her outside she was barely conscious.

An inquiry was unavoidable, and in the circumstances no one tried to avoid one. Eva was suspended pending a report and in the meantime she was interviewed by a forensic psychiatrist. In short order it was established that Eva was ill, and the psychiatrist issued a report saying that Eva could not, at present, be held answerable for her actions. The priority was to find an effective treatment for her.

'She was borderline territory, on paper anyway,' the psychiatrist said. 'She had suffered a physical injury, a brain injury, and her symptoms were consistent with that. But the thing to be borne in mind, from the standpoint of helping her, was that although a strictly physical mishap had created her predicament, the condition was now psychiatric, it was a case of personality-damage that could not be undone by any surgeon. It was up to the shrinks to try and do something for the poor girl.'

While taking a detailed history the psychiatrist discovered that for a couple of weeks Eva had been keeping spectacular secrets from her ever-vigilant sister. Following the one-night event with the biker, Eva had decided two things: she was mad to take him back to their flat, and she was definitely keen to expand her sexual horizons a lot further.

'She had been picking up men with breezy abandon,' the psychiatrist said. 'She couldn't remember how many. And she had done everything imaginable with them, in the sexual sense. She told me she had been having vivid sexual fantasies, and she experienced no qualms or hesitation about carrying them out. That told us a lot, in fact, and not all of it obvious. Eva was displaying signs of what's called the Klüver-Bucy Syndrome, which virtually clinched the diagnosis of temporal-lobe injury. I passed on the information to the appropriate specialists in Hamburg, who had already been alerted to the case and were making arrangements to have Eva admitted to their treatment centre.'

The Klüver-Bucy Syndrome, named for two neurologists who first described it, is a collection of symptoms (impaired memory, rage reactions and hypersexuality among them) that are known to follow injury to the temporal area of the brain in both men and women. Armed with such a clear diagnosis, the therapeutic team were able to map out a relatively precise course of treatment for Eva.

The prognosis in brain-injury cases is not always good. In Eva's case, however, a drug regime was devised which controlled her symptoms so effectively she was able to go back to work within three months.

As the years passed a slow process of healing seemed to be taking place in her brain, and although her cerebral activity would never entirely return to normal, she suffered very few adverse symptoms. She was able to reduce her drug intake, over time, to safe minimal levels. She worked on as a police officer for a further eleven years until she married and emigrated to Australia.

In the ensuing sixteen years no relapse has been reported.

8
Pyromania

'The way I look at it,' a New York police officer said, 'fire-raising is one of the lousiest crimes going. It ought to be punished as severely as murder. The arsonist needs to be discouraged by every means we've got, because that crime is the equivalent of putting a deranged monster in the hands of every inadequate that wants to use one. I'd give arsonists the chair, with no possibility of reprieve.'

Arsonists are difficult to fit into a behaviour category, but a few groups can be identified. First there are the arsonists who suffer from no mental disorder, and who start fires for profit, or to make a political statement; they are sometimes called Motivated Arsonists. The second group are the Pathological Arsonists, who are mentally ill, mentally retarded, or alcoholic. A third group, the ones who concern us here, are said to suffer from Pyromania; they start fires for highly unreasonable motives – for example, to calm some complex inner conflicts, to come to the aid of fire fighters in a daring and courageous way, or to obtain sexual gratification.

The estimates of repetition in arson show there is a high repeat-rate if the fire-raising has an element of fetishism, revenge, paranoid thinking, or 'irresistible impulse'. With all offenders between the ages of 15 and 20 there is an average 30 per cent repeat rate. Among arsonists released from prison, 20 per cent of long-term offenders repeat within 5 years, while in the same period only 2 per cent of short-term offenders repeat their crime.

Freud, not surprisingly, saw fire as a symbol of sexuality. He said the warmth of a fire produces the same voluptuous sensations that accompany sexual excitement, and the dancing flames, furthermore, suggest an active penis. Fire fetishists certainly gain sexual satisfaction from fire-setting, but present-day therapists tend to associate a large proportion of cases of Pyromania with an abnormal craving for power. The disorder is more common among men than women, and as so often happens, it is a subject of disagreement among psychiatrists. Some are convinced it has a group of causes, most of them pathological and in need of sympathetic study, others believe that the behaviour is rooted in sheer malevolence, with no basis in psychiatric illness at all.

Treatment for fire-setters is very difficult, because they do not particularly want to be cured. Often, the only way to be sure of avoiding another episode is to lock the subject up in prison or in a special hospital, where behaviour therapy can be given.

Children who raise fires receive intensive treatment, with the emphasis carefully slanted away from any notion of punishment. Usually the idea is to persuade the child that the act of fire-raising is not desirable, and is in fact rather a dull and boring activity. Careful supervision is needed, however, since some children are adept at pretending they are becoming bored with fire-raising, when in fact the tension towards another episode is steadily building up.

CASE ONE: *The Friend in the Yard*

Although fire-raising is considered by some to be a conduct disorder which goes hand-in-hand with other acts of anti-social behaviour, the subject of this case, André, was known to his family, school friends and teachers as a charming, good-natured boy who fitted well into his domestic and social life. His only flaw was that he kept starting fires.

André was seven when his mother took him to her family doctor at Pontoise, a town north-west of Paris. She was afraid her son would do some serious harm if his fascination with starting fires was not curtailed. She and her husband had done everything in their power to discourage the boy, and they supervised him when they could, but even so he had set a number of fires – two of them rather serious – in the year before he was taken to see the doctor. After examining the boy and finding him healthy, the doctor referred the case to Edouard Barois, a psychiatrist with a weekly clinic at St Denis, on the northern outskirts of Paris.

'I found the boy open and articulate,' Barois said, 'and he seemed almost keen to help me. I took that as a bad sign, since the commonest avoiding-tactic among patients is to welcome the psychiatrist's questions and offer all the help they can give him. However, this was a child, and he had a particularly candid approach, so I reserved judgement and moved forward warily.'

Asked directly why he kept lighting fires, André said he was doing what he was told. 'My friend Luke squeezes my arm, and when he does that I know it's time to light another fire.'

Luke, it transpired, was a semi-visible friend who lived in a corner of the back yard at André's home. Luke was an older boy, a German (André's father was German) who had to be obeyed. There was never any question of refusing him. André explained that he would be killed if he didn't light a fire whenever Luke indicated that he should. It would not be Luke who killed him, he said, it would be somebody, another German and much older, that Luke took orders from.

'I asked André what else Luke told him to do,' Barois said. 'He explained that Luke didn't actually ever *tell* him anything. Luke was a mute, or he behaved like one, and he conveyed everything by contact signals. A squeeze on the arm was a sign to start a fire, a tap on the shoulder meant that André must eat some chocolate, and a pat on top of the head was a sign that it was time to go and play with his friends.'

The psychiatrist tentatively accepted that André believed all this, but when he discussed the interview with André's mother, she said the boy changed his story depending on who he was talking to. Some people, a cousin and André's grandmother, had been given a story about voices in the air above André's head, telling him to burn things. Both his parents were sure that the fires were a form of attack on his father, who was rather strict with the boy and made him quite obviously angry at times.

The early episodes of fire-raising involved outdoor rubbish bins and a garden chair, which André first doused with petrol, then lit with a burning rag thrown at it from a few feet away. Fire appeared to fascinate him: 'The word is mesmerise,' his mother told Barois. 'He stands like somebody entranced, staring at it. He never runs away. If he starts a fire anywhere, you'll always find him standing near it, watching.'

That was what happened when he moved on to larger and more serious targets. He enlisted the help of a friend to pour paraffin on a tool shed in a public park near his home, then he sent the friend away. When several minutes later the shed was seen to be ablaze, the park keeper found André standing nearby, staring as the flames climbed over the roof, setting fire to overhanging tree branches.

'The park keeper was a very practical man,' Barois said. 'He took the view that young villains caught misbehaving in his park would only be given a sharp talking-to if he reported them, and in his view a talking-to was about as much use as an ashtray on a motorbike. So he cuffed André about the ears, took him home and demanded that his father give him a proper hiding. The father demurred, but he thanked the park keeper nevertheless for keeping the matter out of the hands of the authorities.'

The run-in with the park keeper seemed to subdue André for a time, causing his parents to reconsider their view that the corporal punishment of children achieved nothing. However, one afternoon his mother came home to find smoke billowing from an upstairs window. She ran into the house and found André crouched in the doorway of her bedroom, watching the bed burn.

Less than a week after that a neighbour rang André's mother to tell her the greenhouse in the back garden appeared to be on fire. This time there was no sign of the boy, but the greenhouse was blazing from end to end. Later his mother found him in the utility outhouse with a basket of screwed-up paper torches standing by. He admitted that he had first poured paraffin from the butt in the garage over the lower frame of the greenhouse, then lobbed lighted torches at it until it caught fire. He added that he had been told to do this by a man who rang up while his mother was out that morning. The man had added that he would be round to shoot André if he did not do exactly as he was told.

'The act which finally sent his mother in search of professional help was small by comparison to other things André had done,' Barois said, 'but it had the potential for a disaster, and I suppose it frightened her badly. André set light to a duster, then dropped it into the kitchen rubbish bin. At approximately that time a friend called for André and the two went off to play together. The father, asleep upstairs after working a night shift, awoke to the smell of burning. He went downstairs and found the kitchen blackened with smoke which was still pouring from the bin. The family's pet canary was dead in the bottom of its cage. André apparently suffered a lot of unspoken remorse about that, but neither parent believed for a minute that it would stop him lighting more fires.'

The story ended tragically. A month after first meeting Dr Barois, André built a bonfire of paper, dried wood and petrol-soaked rags in precisely the corner of the back yard where he claimed his friend Luke lived. It was a warm day and experts believed that pockets of gas from the petrol had developed within the criss-cross structure of the bonfire. When André put a light to it there was a small explosion, heard several houses away, and the boy was covered in burning fuel. He ran screaming from the yard, his speed fanning the flames, and by the time he fell in the roadway and a neighbour was able to put out the flames with a blanket, the boy had suffered burning to more than three quarters of his body surface. In hospital he was given emergency treatment for the burns and the toxic effects of breathing smoke. He died later that evening.

CASE TWO: *Ecstatic Dreams*

Alessandro is an Italian who studied the finer points of forensic psychiatry in Switzerland and England during the seventies, then returned to practise in Rome in 1982. Since then the tides of opportunity and circumstance, as he puts it, have moved him into a speciality where his diagnostic talent is unquestioned, and his expert evidence for the prosecution in court cases is known to sway juries powerfully, in spite of the best efforts of opposing counsel.

'I specialise in interviewing perverts for the state,' he said. 'In my time here I think I have dealt with every kind of paraphilia – even the *outré* ones like Klismaphilia and Coprophagia.'

For the record, Klismaphilia is a fixation on enemas as a form of sexual excitement; Coprophagia is sexual pleasure from eating faeces.

'It's amazing what a different view you get of these things by dealing with them in real life,' Alessandro said, 'instead of in the pages of the manuals, like the average practitioner has to do. He acquaints himself with *theory*, which is all very tidy. Theory is such a forgiving kind of territory, too. It overlooks the wilfully monstrous and the abominable, it is blind to the calculatingly wicked nature of many people.'

In 1988 Alessandro was asked to interview a suspected fire-raiser on behalf of the police, with a view to assessing the man's state of mind at the time of his alleged crime, and gauging his general fitness to plead. The man was charged with burning down an American-owned import warehouse and causing close to a million dollars' worth of damage. Alessandro was not impressed with the prisoner's physical presence.

'He was the kind of man who has been dirty for so long that even when he has been cleaned up, he tends to exude a stench. He lived on the streets in the southern outskirts of Rome, he scavenged for food and begged for money, and when he needed sexual release, he lit a fire.'

The accused man, Paolo, was thirty-two, a native of

Palermo who had run away from home at the age of fourteen and had not returned since. Until he left home (he
said he did not want any further part of family or social life)
he had been a bright and relatively cheerful boy, though not
particularly intelligent. Living on his own, with no pos-
sessions, he soon deteriorated. For eighteen years he had
lived as a vagrant, attaching himself to groups of street-
dwellers in various cities and towns until coming to Rome
in 1987.

'From time to time he had been admitted to hospitals,'
Alessandro said, 'usually suffering from malnutrition, a
couple of times because he had been beaten up and half-
killed by other street people. In 1979 someone had the
bright idea of fingerprinting him, so some continuity
developed – his records could be verified, we could tell that
the Paolo who drank too much methylated spirit in 1981
was the same Paolo who ate from the wrong dustbin and
almost poisoned himself in 1984.

'From this dossier there emerged a three-page report
made by a psychiatrist who interviewed the prisoner in
1985. Paolo had been in hospital with suspected peritonitis.
He was roped into a survey of homeless people using the
medical services, and by one accident and another, he
wound up telling a psychiatrist about his various weak-
nesses and sad areas.'

Paolo had told the psychiatrist that he dreamed repeatedly about fire; he added that fire was his only love. The
hospital psychiatrist had not pursued that point, but Alessandro did. He quickly learned that Paolo was a classic
fire fetishist.

'He was the second of the only two I've ever met,' Alessandro said, 'and I have to say there was little to choose
between them – solitary, subnormal, withdrawn. Interested

only in scraping by, and having the occasional sexual adventure with a box of matches.'

The fire fetishist has ecstatic dreams about fire and finds his only sexual gratification in mental images, or the reality, of consuming fire.

'Paolo started his career as a fire-raiser when he was fifteen,' Alessandro said. 'He set fire to a hay bale in a field and masturbated as the thing blazed. For a time that was the extent of it, a hay bale here, a hay bale there. Then he fancied trying a barn. He set fire to one in a farmyard in Tuscany, and he got a bonus – a can of petrol or something similar exploded and spread the flames right across the ground in a brilliant, crackling circle. That triggered the best orgasm Paolo had experienced up to that time.'

In the course of revealing his history to Alessandro, Paolo confessed to a number of major acts of arson in and around Rome in the previous eighteen months. In the case of one fire – a restaurant, where a night-watchman died in the blaze – another man was already in prison for the offence.

'In the end it was a mess. I had this man spilling all these details, and the police were beginning to panic, because what he was telling me was cancelling a lot of their certainties and opening up old files again. The amazing part, to me, was that Paolo, a human being like the rest of us, did not care a straw what happened to him. I don't think he had ever cared. When I had the tapes of his talks with me transcribed, a couple of senior police officers spent an afternoon listening to them. They told Paolo afterwards that he would probably go to prison for twenty-five years. He shrugged. It didn't mean anything.'

When the records had been set straight and the important

details of Paolo's testimony verified, the indictment sheet totalled twelve major arson charges. Alessandro testified at Paolo's trial and told the court the prisoner was a degenerate individual with little or no self regard, who burned property simply for the sexual pleasure he derived from watching the destructive power of fire.

The defence asked Alessandro if he was perhaps not being rather medieval in his evaluation of the accused; wasn't degenerate rather an outmoded word? And wasn't Paolo, in fact, suffering from a serious psychiatric disorder?

'Degenerate is far from being an outmoded word,' Alessandro replied, 'and it is a word, furthermore, which fits the prisoner precisely. It means that he has declined in physical and moral properties, he has lost the qualities, qualities he possessed as a boy, which are desirable and proper in civilised men. As for being mentally ill, no, he is not. He has simply done nothing with his mind but treat it with the same neglect he has shown his body. He has regressed, until his appetites are those of a cave dweller.'

Paolo was found guilty of all twelve offences. The judge told him he had been responsible for the destruction of valuable property and human life; he had shown himself to be of no value to his fellow man and scarcely more to himself. He was sentenced to twenty years' imprisonment. On hearing the sentence he nodded curtly and thanked the judge.

CASE THREE: *Imposter*

On a dark, windy evening in late November 1976, Aldo Beckmann, a Pittsburgh bookseller, was counting the cash from his till while his assistant locked up the shop. Pausing by the back door, the assistant said he could smell smoke. Aldo, a notably grumpy and impatient seventy-five-year-old, sniffed the air imperiously, told the assistant he was imagining things, then ordered him to clear off, he would finish locking up by himself.

The assistant had been gone no more than two minutes and was only on the next street when the front of the bookshop exploded and fire raged through the interior. By the time the fire service had brought the blaze under control the body of Aldo Beckmann had been reduced to a charred skeleton.

Eleven days later on 5 December, a Sunday, an elderly woman, Margo Delaney, was asleep on a covered sun balcony behind her home in a suburb of Pittsburgh when the glass-and-wood structure caught fire. She was seen by neighbours trying to open the door, but it was either stuck or locked. Margo was quickly overcome by smoke and she was seen collapsing into the flames. As in the case of Aldo Beckmann the previous month, Margo's body was burned to a skeleton before the fire could be put out.

On 10 December, a man was apprehended by a civilian neighbourhood patrol as he sprayed barbecue fuel on the side of a house on a quiet road towards the south of Pittsburgh. The man struggled but a zealous female member of the patrol team struck him on the head with her heavy-duty torch, subduing him to the point where he needed hospitalisation for concussion.

The police called at the hospital and provisionally booked the injured man, Tom Halliday, a thirty-five-year-old bricklayer, on a charge of attempted arson, and on suspicion of two counts each of arson and murder. The police were confident of making a conviction: fire investigators had determined that barbecue fuel had been used to start the fire at Beckmann's bookshop and at Margo Delaney's house, and footprints found in Margo's side garden matched the soles of the shoes Halliday had been wearing when he was apprehended.

On his third day in hospital Halliday asked to speak to a psychiatrist. Dr Jane Houseman attended, and noted that the patient appeared deeply troubled as he tried to tell her what was on his mind.

'He finally managed to get it out,' she said. 'He told me that since childhood he had been obsessed with fire, with its power and its all-encompassing hunger. That was the language he used, all-encompassing hunger. I asked if he could tell me more, and very haltingly he explained that his only sexual pleasure was from observing fires, preferably serious ones, where masonry came crashing down and sparks filled the air and the glow lit the clouds. He was very graphic in his description. He said that when he saw fires he had to masturbate, and eventually, in order to enjoy arousal and orgasm, he began setting fires himself.'

He went on to tell Dr Houseman that the bookshop fire and the one at the old woman's house had been random pyromaniac bursts, pure impulses that he had been powerless to resist.

'But he added that he didn't know anybody was in those places. He thought they were empty.'

The case against Halliday was now to be complicated by evidence that he was a fire fetishist; a specialist in the management of unusual psychiatric conditions spent several hours talking to Halliday and afterwards agreed to give evidence for the defence. The prisoner, he said, was clearly the victim of a condition which diminished his ability to exercise proper moral judgements. The humane decision of the court would be to send Halliday for a prolonged course of behavioural treatment.

'Three days before the trial was due to start,' Dr Houseman said, 'I had a visit in my office from a woman called Jennifer Halliday. She identified herself as Tom Halliday's sister. She lived in Denver, Colorado, where quite by accident she had seen an out-of-town newspaper report of the arson attacks, and the story about the accused man being a psychotic fire-raiser. She told me that since she read all that, she had felt she was living a crazy nightmare. She saw my name and simply had to come all that way to tell me the truth. None of what the papers said was true.'

It transpired that Tom Halliday was a one-time psychiatric nurse, sacked from his post in a Pittsburgh hospital for stealing money from patients' bedside lockers. It had been a case of his word against the mental patients', and he had taken it hard when the grievance committee chose to believe the patients and sack him.

'He'd had no record, at any time, of fire-fetishism or any other mental illness,' Dr Houseman said. 'But he knew all about the rare mental disorders, his sister said. It had been a hobby with him, or perhaps an unhealthy preoccupation, collecting books and extracts, impressing girlfriends back in Denver with his knowledge of bizarre psychiatric conditions.'

And the knowledge had come to his rescue, or nearly, when he was caught getting ready to set a third fire. The third venue was the home of George Greely, one of the three civilian members of the hospital management subcommittee that had sacked Tom Halliday. The other two members were Margo Delaney and Aldo Beckmann.

'I was taken in by him,' Dr Houseman admitted.

'Me too,' said the specialist. 'He fooled me completely. He had everything just right – the tone of his confession, the content, the air of bewilderment you get with people who are pushed around by their compulsions. If his sister hadn't blown the whistle, I think he might very well have ended up in a comfortable hospital in the hills, soaking up therapy at the taxpayers' expense.'

The psychiatric evidence on Halliday's behalf was withdrawn. He was tried on two counts of arson, two of murder, and one of attempted arson. The jury took one hour to deliberate, then found him guilty. Halliday was sentenced to three terms of life imprisonment.

9
Paranoid Schizophrenia

Schizophrenia comes from two Latin words, *schizo*, meaning to split, and *phren*, the mind, which may have given rise to the widespread and mistaken belief that people suffering from Schizophrenia have split personalities. It would be more accurate to talk in terms of fragmented personality, but in fact Schizophrenia is the most difficult mental disorder to describe accurately. That is largely because so many different psychiatrists, working in many countries, have put forward different concepts of the disease. The attempt here is to be as accurate as possible without being drawn into lengthy or obscure detail, so the following are *broadly* typical illustrations of the acute and chronic phases.

ACUTE SCHIZOPHRENIA
A description of a patient will help demonstrate the main features. Colleagues of a twenty-year-old student nurse noticed that she had begun behaving oddly. At times she would have sudden unexplained fits of anger and claim that

she was being persecuted by senior staff, or by certain
patients; at other times she would laugh secretively for no
obvious reason. As time passed she appeared to be more and
more preoccupied, often staring into space and frowning, as
if she were lost in her own thoughts. Her work began to
deteriorate. When she was eventually questioned by a hospital administrator, she said she knew that her former boyfriend
was conspiring with the local Council to poison the water
supply at her flat. This was being done, she said, in order to
turn her into a Chinese. She was also troubled by voices which
commented on her behaviour, and by strangers loitering in
the hospital corridor who were reading her thoughts.

The case demonstrates the following common features
of Acute Schizophrenia: powerful feelings of being persecuted; a gradual withdrawal from the society of other
people; a decline in work standards; disembodied voices
making comments and criticisms; the belief that other
people can read the subject's mind.

Acute Schizophrenia subjects do not have all these symptoms at the same time; the picture varies widely. In 1973
the World Health Organisation published a list of the most
frequent symptoms of Acute Schizophrenia found in one
major survey. The following is an abbreviated version of
the list.

SYMPTOMS	FREQUENCY (%)
Lack of insight	97
Auditory hallucinations	74
Suspiciousness	66
Voices speaking to the patient	65
Delusional mood	64
Delusions of persecution	64
Thoughts spoken aloud	50

CHRONIC SCHIZOPHRENIA

Thought disorders, sluggish activity, lack of drive, withdrawal and general apathy are typical of the chronic phase. Again, an example will help illustrate the condition.

A man in his late forties lives in a hostel and works for short periods in a charity shop where he is carefully supervised. For years his outward pattern has been the same: he spends most of his time in the hostel alone; he does not bathe regularly or shave or keep himself tidy unless he is prompted to do so. Socially his behaviour is stilted and appears very odd to people who do not know him. He shows no signs of emotion. When he speaks, his voice is slow and flat, and the content of his speech is often vague and incoherent. His behaviour only changes when he has brief acute phases, usually because of some upheaval in the routine at the hostel.

The description above is distinctly typical of the chronic syndrome, which is sometimes called the Schizophrenic Defect State. The most common and noticeable feature is a loss of volition or drive. Initiative disappears. Left alone, the patient stays inactive, or he involves himself in some pointless, repetitive activity. Many patients withdraw to the point where they become completely uncommunicative. The following is a World Health Organisation list of behaviour characteristics in chronic Schizophrenic patients.

CHARACTERISTIC	FREQUENCY (%)
Social withdrawal	74
Under-activity	56
Lack of conversation	54
Few leisure interests	50
Slowness	48
Over-activity	41

Odd ideas	34
Depression	34
Odd behaviour	34
Neglect of appearance	30
Odd postures and movements	25
Threats or violence	23
Poor mealtime behaviour	13
Socially embarrassing behaviour	8
Sexually unusual behaviour	8
Suicidal attempts	4
Incontinence	4

The term Paranoid Schizophrenia indicates that the symptoms of schizophrenia have been reinforced by powerful delusions of persecution, usually coupled to notions of self-importance. Paranoia, on its own, has been described as a tendency to distrust others to a highly abnormal degree.

To be classified as paranoid schizophrenic, a patient must have one or more sharply defined delusions, and/or clearly hear 'voices' talking to him or to each other on a repetitive topic. There must be *no* evidence of incoherence, no sign of flat or 'inappropriate' moods, and no excessive dreaminess or any kind of disorganised behaviour.

It is universally agreed that the paranoid schizophrenic is potentially the most dangerous of all mentally disturbed people.

'From the viewpoint of forensic psychiatry,' said a leading English practitioner, 'Paranoid Schizophrenia is a condition of primary and consuming interest, since it has been the motivating force behind some of the most savage crimes ever committed.'

CASE ONE: *Special Identity*

Beatrice Laing was born in 1960 at Lanark, Scotland, where she was educated and grew up. She had a normal childhood in a stable family; her father was an under-manager at a Motherwell steel works and her mother taught primary-school children in the town of Carluke. Beatrice's brother Derek, three years her junior, eventually became a lecturer in Physics at a local technical college. As a boy Derek was particularly good at sports, and he recalled that when Beatrice was thirteen or fourteen she used to brag to her friends about his ability on the playing field and at track events.

'There was never any jealousy between us, and no serious rivalry that I can remember,' he said. 'In a quiet and I suppose a not-noticeable way, we were as close as any brother and sister could be.'

Beatrice did reasonably well at school and left at seventeen to do secretarial work. She fitted in well at the Council Offices in Hamilton and two years after joining the staff she met Donald Glen, a surveyor, whom she eventually married when she was twenty-two.

'It was all reassuringly harmonious and conventional,' brother Derek recalled. 'Beatrice was doing what was right, it fitted the conventions of the place and the time. She married Donald and they set up home in a bungalow at Netherton, near Motherwell. The only sour note was when they discovered, two years after they were married, that Beatrice had tubal problems and they couldn't have children.'

The couple continued to work and kept up a moderately busy social life until three and a half years into the marriage, when Beatrice began to feel intermittently depressed and anxious. She saw her doctor a few times, and as the symptoms grew worse she was referred to a psychiatrist, who diagnosed depressive illness. Beatrice was treated with anti-depressants, but she appeared to get no better. She lost her confidence and much of her self-esteem, and finally could no longer do her job.

Two months after Beatrice left the Council Offices her husband, Donald, was assigned by his company to a project in the United States. Beatrice was visibly cheered by the prospect of spending time in America, but a few weeks after they settled into their quarters in Buffalo, New York, she became acutely psychotic and suffered delusions that she was in serious trouble with the US authorities. She became confused and withdrawn and was finally sent back to Scotland, where she was immediately hospitalised.

Eventually a diagnosis was made: the record said Psychiatric Illness (Possibly Schizophrenia). Beatrice remained in hospital for several months, during which time her husband completed his stint in America and returned to Scotland. He found it very difficult to cope with the situation as it now stood. Beatrice was released from hospital, but had to be readmitted, twice, when her delusional symptoms flared up again. Finally Donald left her.

Beatrice moved in with her mother at their old home in Lanark. In old age the mother, a widow by now, was domineering and inclined to nag. She exercised a superficial control over Beatrice, who filled her time by visiting the public library, shopping and working on a series of tapestries. She defaulted on her psychiatric care for six months, during which time her brother Derek kept up a tenuous contact with her and his mother.

Derek became concerned when Beatrice started acting coldly towards him on his visits, treating him like an unwelcome guest and all but asking him to leave when he had been in the house for only a few minutes.

'She definitely underwent a personality change,' he said later. 'She had never been a hard person, or even remotely tough, but now she had this glint in her eye, and she responded very coldly to my questions and never asked any herself. My mother still tried to push her around, but Beatrice didn't take any notice. She just glanced at the old woman from time to time as if she was an old dog that might misbehave and needed to be watched.'

The steely vigilance was not restricted to the mother, Derek noticed.

'I was painfully aware she hardly ever blinked when she spoke to me, as if she was watching for some kind of false move and didn't want to miss it. I felt all the time like I was under suspicion. Then one morning I called round and the door was locked. I tried to use my key but the lock had been changed. Beatrice answered the door and she had this wild look in her eye. She looked angry about something.'

Derek also noticed that she was uncharacteristically dishevelled looking, and her eyes were deep set and red rimmed, as if she hadn't slept. She refused to let Derek into the house and finally slammed the door in his face.

He went back next day, because he was concerned about both his mother and Beatrice. This time when Beatrice answered the door she was openly hostile and brandished a carving knife at her brother.

'I'd never heard her swear, not once in her life,' he said. 'Now she told me to fuck off, and then she slammed the door shut.'

Derek went to the neighbours to ask if they had seen anything of his mother. He was told there had been a lot of noise from the house – hammering and banging, hysterical shouting and the sound of crockery breaking. During the night, one woman said, Beatrice had begun throwing items of household furniture out of a bedroom window into the garden. There had also been the sounds of Beatrice and her mother arguing loudly with each other.

Derek called the police. Two officers went to his mother's front door and knocked sharply. Beatrice appeared at once and threatened both policemen with the carving knife. They retreated and called for reinforcements. Ten minutes later a number of officers wearing body armour broke down the door and stormed inside. Beatrice, a large and powerfully built woman, went berserk and attacked them. The police withdrew again, unsure how to proceed.

'I've warned you!' Beatrice screamed at them from a window. 'You were told! This will be all your doing!'

With that she strode into the kitchen where her mother was hiding. She locked the door, then stabbed her mother forty times in the stomach with the carving knife.

Hearing the screams the police ran back to the house and broke down the kitchen door. Beatrice was leaning by the sink, her arms folded. Her mother lay dead at her feet in a pool of blood.

Beatrice was taken into custody and put in a secure cell at a remand centre. She was interviewed by a psychiatrist who found her to be acutely psychotic.

'She harboured the delusion that her brother and the neighbours had formed a plot against her,' the psychiatrist said. 'She told me they resented the fact that she was really the illegitimate child of a senior member of the Royal family. They wanted to deprive her of her birthright. The neighbours, she said, had pumped gas through the walls in an effort to take away her memory and make her forget who she really was. The arrival of the police confirmed her suspicion that she was being attacked because of her special identity. She believed that her mother had somehow managed to summon the police, and for something so wicked she deserved to be punished. Beatrice had felt no qualms about using the knife on the old woman.'

A forensic psychiatrist had to determine whether Beatrice was fit to plead in court. In making the determination, he had to ask himself five questions, bearing in mind that it was the state of her mind at the time of going to court that mattered in this instance, and not her mental state when she committed her crime.

Q. *Did the accused understand the charge against her, and its possible consequences?*

A. Beatrice could not be convinced that she had done anything which merited punishment. It was the others who were wicked, and they should all pay the price as her mother had.

Q. *Did she understand the difference between a guilty and a not-guilty plea?*

A. She did not recognise the court, which in her view was an extension of the conspiracy to rob her of her birthright.

Q. *Could she instruct a legal representative?*

A. Not at all, since she did not believe there was any charge to answer, besides which lawyers were in on the plot, too, whether they said they were acting for Beatrice or not.

Q. *Would she be able to follow the evidence in court?*

A. No, because she was attached to a separate

'reality' and could not relate to the details of the charge against her.

Q. *Could she challenge a juror?*
A. Only on the grounds that she believed he or she was one of the conspirators.

Beatrice was considered entirely unfit to plead – the phrase used was 'under disability'. She was eventually installed in a secure psychiatric unit, where she withdrew swiftly into apathy and non-communication. She is still there, and she has not changed.

CASE TWO: *A Saviour for our Times*

'I can't ignore the signs and the messages,' Lewis Briggs told his girlfriend. 'I knew a long time ago I was special. But as time's gone by I've felt a powerful truth swelling inside me, warning me I'm more than maybe I suspected. I've been told I have to prepare myself for the truth. I have to be strong and carry the weight of my responsibility.'

Lewis was a twenty-six-year-old gym instructor working for a private health club in Los Angeles. His girlfriend Carla worked for the same club as a receptionist. She reported Lewis's remarks to her doctor, whose husband, she knew, was a psychiatrist. She was very intense and obviously needed to talk to someone who understood mental disturbance; the doctor spoke to her husband, and within a week Carla was invited to visit the psychiatrist and tell him more about it.

'It worries me the way Lewis goes on,' she said. 'For hours on end I can't concentrate on my work for worrying. He's so intense when the moods are on him, and he gets a faraway look, like one of those creepy TV evangelists. He never used to be like this, talking all crazy. It comes and goes, for days he won't say anything weird at all, then it'll be back, he'll say things like, "I was told to build up my strength, I'll need it soon more than I've ever needed it before." And when I ask him who told him that, he says it was a voice of someone close, someone who probably was there all along.'

The psychiatrist asked Carla to keep in touch, since he guessed (accurately) that he was getting a first-hand account of a developing case of Paranoid Schizophrenia. A week later Carla was back at his office. Lewis Briggs, she announced, had finally flipped.

'He says he's Jesus Christ.'

The psychiatrist had already encountered a few messiahs in Los Angeles, a town which seems to attract uncanny numbers of people who believe they are some distance above the ordinary. He pressed Carla for details.

'The word came to him when he was out jogging,' she said. 'He came back to the apartment looking all awe-struck, you know, amazed, like somebody that'd had incredible news. Which he had, of course. A voice, a particular one he's been hearing a lot, told him he's Jesus. He's Jesus and he's got a mission, he'll get the details later. I said, "Lew, this is crazy," and he just smiled at me, like that was what he'd expected me to say.'

The psychiatrist asked Carla if she could list the ways Lewis had changed from the man she first knew.

'He's just about as different as he could get,' she said. 'He looks the same, in his features and his build, but even that's turned strange, because he carries himself peculiarly, and he has a different expression. He walks like there's broken glass all over and he has to walk carefully or he'll cut himself, and he gets this grim, faraway look like he's wearing a Walkman, except he never uses one. And he's given up sex.'

It took only a few more questions for the psychiatrist to form the opinion that this development displeased Carla more than anything else – certainly to the extent that she was now openly considering leaving Lewis. He had sat down with her, holding her hands, and explained that being Christ was a state of purest grace. It was a revelation as much to him as it was to her, but now that he knew who he was, there were certain things he had to change.

'No sex, no red meat, no rock music in the apartment, and no alcohol – just a little red wine, and then only occasionally.'

The psychiatrist asked Carla for her candid opinion of what was happening. Did she feel, perhaps, that Lewis might be putting her on?

'No, not at all. I would know if he tried that. I know him top to bottom, there's no way he could lie and get it past me. I'm sure Lewis truly believes he is Jesus Christ and he's genuinely getting ready for the tasks ahead, whatever they are.'

So how did she feel about him now, deep down?

'For a while I thought what the hell, he's going through a crazy phase, it could be an acid backlash, he used to dabble with the stuff, but now what I feel is . . .'

The psychiatrist reported that at this point Carla began, quite unexpectedly, to cry. He let her recover in her own time, and when she did she said, 'What I feel is that he's slipped out of himself, out of his body, and some joker's got in. That's not what it is, I know that, but that's exactly how it feels to me. He's definitely different, all over. That's the truth, it's as if he had been scooped out of himself and a substandard or goofy version stuck in there in his place.'

People living close to individuals with schizophrenic disorders often report how changed they become, how they appear to be faulty replicas of themselves. Carla said that even in sleep Lewis Briggs had changed, his facial tensions were different, and even his breathing pattern had changed.

'Now that I know this stuff is on his mind all the time, I can tell he's preoccupied even though he pretends not to be. He'll throw up his job next. That'll be it, you wait and see. He can't afford to do that, but he'll do it just the same.'

And did Carla really think she would leave Lewis?

'I believe I'm close to doing that,' she said.

Three days later Lewis told his employer he was leaving. He gave no reason, beyond saying he had important work to do and the gym would get in the way of his doing it. Carla returned to their apartment in the evening to find Lewis sitting in the kitchen wearing a new white tracksuit and snow-white trainers. He was drinking herb tea, a recently acquired taste, and reading from a Good News Bible open on the table in front of him. He looked up and smiled at Carla as she came in. It was a hard smile, she recalled, not as gentle as his smiles had been in the last week or so. It reminded her, she said, of the way a certain bully used to smile when she and her young brother had to walk past him on the way to school.

'Lewis told me to sit down,' Carla told the psychiatrist. 'He said he had been given his mission, and it was a big one just like he had expected. It was a job that had to be carried out once every eighty years when Christ came back. He was in Los Angeles for a reason, he said, and the reason was that the agents of Satan had gathered here. They move about, he says, they set up headquarters where they think it's safe and they won't be noticed, then they multiply and spread their evil.'

Lewis had been told how to identify the Satanic agents, but he couldn't tell Carla since the information was privileged. It was at this point Carla told Lewis she was leaving him.

'He laughed and said I couldn't do that. He needed me. I told him tough shit, but he grabbed hold of me – he's never done that before, he held me so tight he bruised my arm – and he told me I would do what I was told. I got really pissed off at him and I said what about all that gentle Jesus stuff? How come if he was Our Lord he was manhandling me like this? And he smiled again, that hard-looking grin, and he says, "I'm a Saviour for our times!"'

Carla had not yet left him, she said, because she was frankly scared. The psychiatrist told her it might be a good idea to go somewhere safe for a while, perhaps out of town, but she said that wasn't practical, she had to keep her job, so Lewis would always know where to find her. She promised to be careful, and said she did not think it would be a good idea if she came to see the psychiatrist for a while, since she had half an idea that Lewis was watching her.

The psychiatrist had been passing on details of his sessions with Carla to a colleague, a forensic psychiatrist called Edgar Brent. Two days after the last reported meeting with Carla, Dr Brent was asked by the police to make an evaluation of a white male they had in their custody. It was Lewis Briggs.

'He was a formidable looking man,' Brent reported, 'over six feet, blond, muscular, with very steady blue eyes. He was in a holding cell being guarded by two police officers. He had been arrested two hours before for assault on three white males and for causing extensive damage to no fewer than sixteen automobiles.'

At first Lewis said he did not want to talk to Dr Brent who, for all Lewis knew, was one of *them*.

'One of who?'

'If you're one of them, you'll know who. If you're not, you don't need to know.'

'But you can't tell if I'm one of them or not?'

This seemed to present Lewis with a problem, as Dr Brent had assumed it would. Lewis was, after all, the Messiah. All things were known to him.

'The Devil has his powers too,' Lewis finally said.

Dr Brent took that to mean that Lewis believed Satan and his agents could fool the Saviour, if they chose to.

'I promise you,' Dr Brent told Lewis, 'I'm not one of them. I only want to help.'

Lewis thought about that, and while he was thinking he was brought a cup of herbal tea and that seemed to put him in a less confrontational frame of mind. He shrugged at Dr Brent.

'Can I ask you, Lewis, why you attacked those men?'

'They're agents of darkness, enemies of the true light.'

'How do you know they are?'

'They have a green aura. It's visible to the righteous, unless they deliberately hide it.'

'And the cars? Why did you take an axe to so many cars?'

'They're green,' Lewis replied.

Dr Brent looked at the police officers and they looked at each other. One of them went into the corridor and called the desk. When he came back he was able to confirm that all sixteen of the cars attacked by Lewis had green bodywork.

'It was the colour that made you attack them?' Dr Brent said.

Lewis said yes, it was. 'The agents of darkness have green cars. It's how they know each other in the daylight.'

'But surely other people have green cars? Ordinary people?'

'Not around here they don't,' Lewis said.

At the formal indictment Dr Brent advised the court that further examination of the prisoner would be advisable, since one brief interview had already indicated he might be suffering from a serious mental disorder. The judge fixed a date for a hearing and asked Dr Brent to prepare a report on Lewis Briggs's mental state, and to determine his fitness to plead.

Six hours of interview established that Lewis was a full-blown paranoid schizophrenic. His belief that he was Jesus Christ had hardened since his arrest. 'Adversity suited the role,' said Dr Brent. 'He was being victimised for trying to fight the good fight. Who could be more Christ-like than somebody in that situation?'

A major fear plaguing Lewis at this point was his failure even to get under way with his big mission. He could not expect special immunity, he said, not when he was opposing the Devil's people, who could cancel divine immunity simply by concentrating on it – 'But I would have thought I'd make some mark on them, cut down their numbers by a half or more . . .'

Dr Brent asked if Lewis had intended to kill the agents of Satan.

'No. They can't be killed. But they can be neutralised.'

'How?'

'By the mark of the cross, hammered into their flesh.'

An odd feature of the assaults was suddenly clear. Lewis had used a short-handled hammer with a head chiselled almost to a point, then flattened off at the tip, which was cross-shaped. It had been assumed the hammer, a crude-looking implement, had been the nearest thing to hand when Lewis had set out to attack his victims. Questioned now by Dr Brent, he confirmed that he had made it specially for the task, even though he had no particular skills as a tool maker.

Rounding off the final interview, Dr Brent asked Lewis how he felt now about his girlfriend, Carla. Did he still feel the affection for her that had brought them together in the first place?

'She's betrayed me by her lack of faith,' Lewis replied. 'She's the whole cause and reason for my heaviest penance.'

'You have to do penance?'

'I certainly do. I'm God's son, I'm not God. I have to ask my father's forgiveness for my errors.'

'And can't you in your turn forgive Carla?'

'The way the divine law stands now, there is no forgiveness. But in my heart I was weak enough to forgive her for doubting me and for trying to leave me. I have to do penance for that mistake every night.'

'And what would you do, if you were in a position to put right your mistake with Carla?'

'I would kill her,' Lewis said. 'That's the law, now. It's a harsh law. These times need harsh remedies.'

With prompting he added that Carla could never be forgiven, because it wasn't in her heart or her nature to acknowledge the true light. So, Dr Brent asked, was that it? Did Carla remain under sentence of death?

'Definitely.'

On Dr Brent's recommendation Lewis Briggs was committed to a secure psychiatric hospital. During his third month there his condition deteriorated and he appeared to withdraw into a chronic phase, which persisted, and now varies only occasionally when there are changes in his routine or in his surroundings. There are no foreseeable plans to have Lewis released into the community.

CASE THREE: *Cutting Out the Badness*

Religious obsession is often a central feature of schizophrenic disorder, usually because the obsessive temperament seeks goals that are hard to achieve and which, once achieved, are difficult to maintain.

'Many obsessive types will throw themselves into disciplines which promise to show them in their true spiritual form, with all its pocks and pustules,' said Dr Frieda Bruch, a German forensic psychiatrist. 'So many of these people are set on demeaning themselves, to prove there are grounds for their instinctive self-loathing.'

Dr Bruch related the case of Otto, nineteen, a language student who in his second year at university began to show signs of withdrawal, and confided to a girlfriend (a relationship he soon afterwards broke off) that he was sure other students were listening to his thoughts. At mid-term he dropped out of university and went to Dresden, where he used half his savings to pay a year's advance rent on an attic room overlooking a church.

Soon Otto was to be seen in the church in the mornings, sitting silently, hands clasped in his lap, staring at the stained-glass window above the altar. His afternoons appeared to be spent in a public library. Later, a library assistant told police officers that Otto always read from the same three books – *Reverence for Life* by Albert Schweitzer, *A History of Religious Ideas* by Mircesa Eliade, and *The Courage to Be* by Paul Tillich. She added that he made extensive notes from each of the books.

Otto's landlady said he never brought friends back to his room, and he seemed to go to bed early most nights. He never went out in the evening.

In the main, Otto attracted little attention to himself, and those who took any notice of him assumed he was just a quiet, studious, religiously-inclined young man.

But inwardly Otto was seething. A general practitioner was the first to know about this when Otto visited him and asked for something to help him sleep. The doctor questioned him about his sleeplessness and discovered Otto was kept awake by voices. Every night, as soon as he had put out the light and lain down, voices began to speak to each other, seemingly in the room where he lay; they talked about what he had learned that day and how his understanding of religion was progressing and, more importantly, how well he was doing in his efforts to be a good man.

'There was a central conflict,' the doctor reported, 'a belief that he must be a good and pure man, a virtual saint, and this belief was in direct opposition to his normal appetites and inclinations.'

The voices told about Otto's failure. They ridiculed him and said what a loser he was, what a weak, spineless, insipid excuse for a man of God, who couldn't keep his mind off women long enough to learn the disciplines of the upright Christian life.

'Secretly, without anyone in his lodging house knowing, he crept out two nights a week, sometimes three,' the doctor said. 'He would go to a red-light district, pick up a prostitute, and pay her for a really extravagant couple of hours of sex.'

In this way Otto hoped to rid himself of his sexual needs, which he firmly believed were unworthy of his true nature, which he saw himself as excavating from a welter of worldly filth.

'He suffered greatly over this trade with the prostitutes,' the doctor said. 'He was tormented by it. I encouraged him to visit me regularly, to see if we couldn't resolve his conflicts, or at least reduce them. But he seemed to get worse. He would spend a whole night with one or two whores, crawl home exhausted – 'cleansed' was what he called it – and immerse himself in his devotional studies, feeling himself to be clean and close to a state of grace, until the sexual itch started up again. And of course, the more he got up to with the prostitutes, in an effort to purge himself of his appetites, the stronger his appetites grew. I tried to explain that to him, that he was exercising his libido and giving it muscles, but he didn't want to hear me. He had formed his own ideas about what was happening and he wouldn't accommodate common sense.'

The doctor coaxed Otto to visit a psychiatrist and he eventually agreed, telling the doctor he was only doing it because a psychiatrist would be likely to have a sympathetic ear, if Jung was anything to go on.

'He came to my consulting rooms four times,' the psychiatrist said. 'He was keen to lecture me, in his quiet way. He needed help, he said, to formulate a means whereby he could suppress his sexual appetites and achieve two important goals – one, to lead a blameless life of the spirit, so that he would be pure enough in heart to commune daily with Christ, and two, to finally shut up the nagging voices. By now, he had decided he mustn't use drugs to induce sleep or reduce his sexual drive. It all had to be done through sheer strength of mind and toughness of will. He said he was sure I could help him.'

The psychiatrist's main objective, at that stage, was to get a firm diagnosis. He was pretty sure that Otto was schizophrenic, but not sure enough. At the second and third visits he tried to elicit more information about the voices, and about Otto's recent belief that he was being controlled from within by a small, hot core of 'badness'.

'He believed he had been overcoming his weakness, and then the badness had been implanted deliberately to set back his progress,' the psychiatrist said. 'I tried to get him to explain the badness. He said it was like a spiritual cancer, a presence in his own body that was designed to undermine every good intention and every fine ambition. When I asked him where he thought it had come from, he would only say he had his suspicions.'

On the fourth visit to the psychiatrist Otto announced this would be the last time they would meet. He thanked the doctor for his kindness and for the time he had made available, but since he now believed nothing was to be gained by the meetings, there was no sense in keeping them going.

'I couldn't change his mind. He thanked me again and left.'

Two days later, Otto was arrested at his lodgings and taken to the police station, where he was formally charged with causing serious bodily harm to a prostitute.

'I meant to kill her,' he told Dr Bruch, who was the forensic psychiatrist appointed by the authorities to assess Otto's mental state. When she asked why he had wanted to kill the woman, Otto said, 'It was the appropriate action.'

For the next two days he refused to say anything more. He was transferred to a secure psychiatric facility, where he told another prisoner that the prostitute had put an implant into him, a core of badness, and that she would do it to someone else if she wasn't stopped. He was deeply sorry that he had not managed to kill her, though he appeared to brighten when he was told that following her release from hospital, the woman had suffered a relapse and was found to be suffering from a cerebral haematoma.

'Perhaps she'll die after all,' Otto remarked.

After three days in the secure facility he began to show signs of withdrawal. He would speak to no one and sat always where he could look through a window and ignore the others around him. He asked to be allowed to stay in his cell during the day; the authorities were happy to accommodate him, since the arrangement meant he was one less prisoner to watch during communal sessions in the games room and workshops.

On the sixth day of his detention Otto put a sheet of paper over the spy hole in his cell door so that no one could look in. A guard noticed it at mid-morning and quickly opened the cell door. He recalled being frozen in the doorway, shocked by what he saw. Otto sat naked in the corner on the stone floor by the window. He was sitting in a pool of blood. In his hand he held a razor blade, and in front of him on the floor were his testicles, cut into neat slices.

He was rushed to the infirmary, where emergency surgery stopped the haemorrhage and transfusions pulled him back from the brink of death. After he recovered, a number of days passed before he would speak to anyone. When Dr Bruch arrived he agreed to see her.

'I was told where the badness was planted,' he explained to her. 'A sacrifice was needed, and the same sacrifice would ensure my salvation. Which it did. The badness was cut out and the slicing destroyed it. I would never have let it spread.'

Some time later the secure unit reported that Otto was announcing contact with Vikings, who had provisionally agreed to impart the secret of immortality. Since it looked as if another sacrifice might be the price of this new wisdom, a close watch was being kept on the patient, who was also being treated with tranquillisers, against his wishes.

'Otto had moved further away from reality each time I saw him,' Dr Bruch said. 'In the end the diagnosis was paranoid schizophrenia. As if to underscore that, the very morning I co-signed the order having him indefinitely committed, he told a male nurse that he was going to report him to the administration for stealing his thoughts. An hour later he tried to suffocate the nurse by throwing him down, sitting on his chest and jamming a balled-up pair of socks into his mouth, then poking them halfway down his throat.'

CASE FOUR: *Devil in the Ear*

Kate was an attractive twenty-one-year-old native of Milwaukee where she worked in a small factory stringing tennis racquets. She came from a disrupted family background (father frequently absent, mother alcoholic and violent) and Kate had spent a number of years in care. At the age of eighteen she came out of care and drifted for a time, doing various menial jobs to make enough money to last her a week at a time. She never held a job for longer than ten days and never had a permanent place to live until at the age of nineteen she met a woman who was a member of the Children of Grace, a fairly isolationist religious group; the woman talked to Kate for a long time and, in Kate's own words, her life changed. She joined the sect and became firmly attached to them.

A man called Edgar who had authority in the local group arranged for Kate to have a job in the tennis racquet factory, and he found her a small two-room apartment, which his wife Donna helped Kate to furnish. Kate became very close to this couple; there was a suspicion of a sexual link between her and the man, although he denied it.

Kate had no history of psychiatric illness, but about six

months after she had joined the Children of Grace, and
over only a period of days, she began to behave oddly,
looking very distracted, failing to respond when people
spoke to her, and becoming noticeably more attached to her
Bible, which she seemed to be reading at every opportunity.

A girl at the factory tried to find out what was wrong.
She spoke to Kate at the lunch break and asked her if
anything was getting her down.

'The Devil is tempting me,' Kate said. The other girl was
too embarrassed to ask any more. Kate sat staring at her
for a while, then she said, 'He gets in through my ear. It's
different with everybody, with me it's the left ear. He makes
me think terrible things.'

A few days later the female manager at the factory heard
Kate talking in the toilet. Later the same day she heard her
in there talking again. The next time Kate went to the toilet,
there was a microphone slung over the top of the cubicle
and the manager tape-recorded what the girl said. The tape
later came into the possession of the police; on it, Kate
whispered urgently as if she were in face-to-face contact
with someone who could help her, but the language she
spoke was from another century.

'Incline thine ear unto my calling,' she whispered. 'My
soul is full of trouble and my life draweth nigh unto hell. I
am counted as one of them that go down into the pit, and
I have been even as a woman that has no strength . . .'

A psychiatrist with theological training was able, later,
to throw an interesting light on this. The words, he said,
were from the Psalms as they were translated in the King
James Version of the Bible. But the Children of Grace use
their own translation. A little research was able to uncover
the fact that during her early teen years, while she was
in care, Kate was a keen Bible student and was trained in

Scripture by a Presbyterian minister who was chaplain to the home where she was cared for at that time.

'There could have been a conflict of loyalties here,' the psychiatrist said, 'although she never indicated that any existed. However, she denied an association with the Presbyterians, and we know that isn't true, so something was covered up, and it was probably to do with a clashing of principles – for instance, she could have felt a sentimental attachment for her earlier religious conviction, but was emotionally drawn to the new one, which demanded she reject all others.'

Whatever the case, Kate's behaviour became stranger as time passed. She communicated less and appeared to be talking to herself as she worked. At Children of Grace services in the local meeting hall she impressed others with the energetic way she assimilated the sect's messages and demonstrated her determination to learn more. Everyone noticed that she seemed particularly attached to Edgar and Donna, but within the group, at that time, her behaviour gave no cause for curiosity or concern.

Approximately ten days after the factory manager had taped Kate's prayer in the toilet, there was a noisy scene on the street outside the factory which ended with the police being called. Kate had been standing just outside the door putting on her coat, when a man going past said something to his companion that infuriated Kate.

'Massey is just an idiot,' the man said.

The next thing he knew Kate had hit him with her umbrella and pushed him against a telegraph pole, where she held him with one hand clamped on his throat.

'Pastor Massey is in Heaven!' she screamed at him. 'He was a good man and people just spread filthy lies about him!'

Later, when peace had been restored, Edgar came to take Kate home from the police station. He explained that Pastor Massey was the byname of David Desmond Massey, the founder of the International Association of Bible Scholars, from which the Children of Grace was an outgrowth. There had been rumours in Massey's lifetime about marital infidelity, and there had been lawsuits, one of them surrounding Massey's alleged embezzlement of charity funds. Kate had read a lot about Pastor Massey in recent times, Edgar told the police, so her response to what the bypasser said was no more than a misunderstanding. The police were happy to let Kate go, but a female officer remarked prophetically, 'She'll be back.'

Now the Children of Grace themselves began to notice that Kate was behaving oddly. There was nothing natural in her reactions to the presence of other people, she behaved robotically and in an over-mannered way, as if she had to think of a response and marshal it carefully before she put it into action.

'She stopped making herself attractive, too,' said a woman who worked with her. 'She was a real good-looker, men always took notice, but she began playing it down, she stopped wearing make-up and she let her hair get in a mess. If any guy looked at her she turned aside real sharply, as if he had spat at her.'

Early one Friday morning, before work had started, when the women were sitting at their benches talking, waiting for the eight-thirty bell, Kate appeared and threw down a magazine in front of one of the women. It was folded open at a nude picture of a grinning blonde.

'Slut!' Kate said, and flounced away to her own bench.

The women all looked at each other. The picture was nothing like the woman Kate had called a slut, apart from the hair colour. As they were starting work a few minutes later, one woman said she would talk to the manager about that oddball.

But Kate left the factory after only an hour, before anybody had time to lay a complaint. She made no explanation. She simply got her coat and went. An hour later she was seen by a neighbour arriving at the home of Edgar and Donna. Donna answered the door and showed Kate in.

'It was maybe five minutes after that,' the neighbour told police, 'I saw her come out again, and she had blood on her face and on her beige coat, and it was on the fronts of her legs too in long streaks, and she just as casual as you like came across the lawn on to the sidewalk and wandered up the road, as if she didn't have a care in the world.'

The neighbour called the police. When they went into the house where Kate had been they found Donna lying dead in the kitchen. Her throat had been cut and one eye had been gouged out. Kate was arrested less than a mile away, strolling through a shopping mall, apparently oblivious to the fact that she was covered in blood and attracting the shocked attention of other shoppers. A psychiatrist pointed out later that people who kill as a result of acute psychosis feel they have done something rational, and therefore take no particular steps to avoid the consequences of their action.

Kate was declared to be a paranoid schizophrenic, and unfit to plead. Although she was questioned at length she gave no reason for killing Donna, although she agreed that she had done it, and had meant to do it. Edgar assured the police that he could throw no light on the mystery, and insisted that his relationship with Kate had never been less than proper.

CASE FIVE: *Voices*

The case of David, a junior staff member in a bank in Manitoba, Canada, has curious echoes of Otto's history, not least in the part played by a razor in resolving a conflict.

David joined the bank when he was seventeen and was popular with customers and other members of staff.

'A regular Mr Sunshine,' was how his manager described him. 'He was living proof that a warm smile can melt a cold heart. We used to encourage him to deal with our grouchy customers, and he never failed to get a good response out of them. David did excellent PR for this branch, and he did it without having to try.'

David played squash in his spare time, had a semi-serious relationship with a girl his own age who was training to be a teacher, and maintained a link with his old school through sports programmes and social events.

'Locally he was an icon,' said a forensic psychiatrist, Dr Loomis. 'People were pleased to be known by him. He was handsome and fair-haired, naturally graceful, a white-teethed Adonis. He amounted to a stereotype for healthy, good-living, forward-looking youth. The image was miles too good to be true.'

What David did best was cover up his real nature. He was beset by fears and conflicts, a constant prey to uncertainty about his right to exist, and about his eventual fate.

'I was sure, quite often, that I was on the verge of death,' he told Dr Loomis. 'I used to be able to see the pulse at my wrist. I would stare at it, beating there, so fragile, and I would think in a panic how unlikely it was that it would keep doing that. It looked to me like it might quit any second.'

The fear of imminent death was intermittent; there were times when it did not trouble David at all. On the other hand his attraction to other males was never dormant, and neither was his guilt.

'He was amphigenic,' Dr Loomis said, 'which is to say he was attracted to both sexes.'

Bisexual is not a term to encourage, Dr Loomis added; it is hard to employ accurately now, because it gets used in so many different ways, from indicating men and women with the mental attributes of the opposite sex, to representing indulgence in both heterosexual and homosexual behaviour.

'David was drawn almost as much by women as men, but he suffered a lot of conflict over his attraction to his own sex, therefore it assumed a large and disproportionate significance in his daily life.'

In his first six months with the bank David was propositioned by a visiting director and later spent two days with the man at his weekend home in the country. Afterwards he experienced powerful guilt about the event and refused to see the older man again.

'It was the way I lied to my girlfriend, and to my parents,' he told Dr Loomis. 'It really got to me. I knew people liked me and trusted me, and the people near to me really put *total* trust in me. Yet I could do that, I could lead the kind of double life that they would hate in another person, and I could lie to them, smiling, so that I could carry out the deceit.'

Dr Loomis was impressed with David's talent for analysing his situation and his motives, especially since the circumstances that brought David to the interviews were classically psychotic and deranged. But before any of that happened, David was being drawn into another area of conflict.

'If I'd heard about anybody else in my place doing it, I

would have said, well, he's a fool, a damn fool and he should get caught, just so he learns a valuable and necessary lesson.'

David stole some money. He took it to solve a family problem arising from his grandmother's need for a motorised wheelchair, now that his grandfather was dead and there was no one to push her around the house and to do the shopping.

'It was a corny scenario, but there was the potential in it for tragedy,' said Dr Loomis, 'because the old lady was getting despondent, what with being stuck so far away from her family, with no real friends, and her only form of contact with the world being taken away. David felt her sense of isolation keenly, and he knew what would solve it. Money. And every day he worked with piles of the stuff.'

To his family David made it appear that he had been able to organise a loan at special staff rates, but he added that it had been done only semi-officially, since he had not been with the bank long enough to qualify officially, so he asked them to say nothing about the loan to anyone outside.

The theft caused David terrible guilt which was intensified, he believed, by the fact that no one detected it. The money, $3,000, had been taken from a floating amount carried in a special till, and somehow the computer had bypassed the amount in its calculations of the till's end-of-week balance.

'David believed that if there had at least been a danger of him being caught,' Dr Loomis said, 'the jeopardy would have been some measure of redress for his crime, and he would not have felt so bad. As matters stood he felt, so he said, as if something hard and heavy were positioned squarely across his shoulders, weighing him down, and he could think of nothing without his brain seeming to ache.

In short, he was suffering extreme guilt. His mind was under assault from many directions. In my view, he was wide open for psychosis.'

The first signs came two days after David had deceived his girlfriend again. He had cancelled their date and gone off to meet a man who had literally picked him up while he was conducting a cash transaction at the bank counter. It was done swiftly and the man had passed the address of a restaurant through the security tray to David. The rendezvous began with a pleasant meal but ended badly in a hotel room, when the man's fetishistic demands scared David and he had to beat him off before making his escape.

'Two days later it came to David that he must interpret a sign that was being given to him right there in the bank, by an old lady looking for something in her purse,' Dr Loomis said. 'He was convinced that although she was right across the other side of the bank, and not even looking at him, she knew all about him and his conflicts, and was making signs that he must decode if he was to make sure the rest of the day passed without disaster enveloping him.'

The message, David believed, was that he must have no lunch break, and that he must volunteer for the least pleasant jobs going at tidy-up time after the bank's doors closed. He did this gladly, and felt better afterwards.

'At that stage it was a kind of obsessive-compulsive thing,' Dr Loomis said. 'From day to day he would imagine he was getting signs that he must first interpret, then act upon, and really, they were no more than small acts of penance for being the bad person he believed he was. But this stage was transitional and pretty harmless. It wasn't long before he began hearing voices.'

David heard the first one when he was sitting watching

television with his girlfriend. At first he thought it was on the TV; it said, *They've got David and they're really going to make him suffer.* He looked at his girlfriend and asked her what that had meant. She didn't know what he was talking about, she had heard nothing unusual. A few minutes later he was in the kitchen making coffee and the same voice said, *They'll pull him down and get him ready for destruction.* A second voice then added, *The ridiculous thing is he'll love it, he's so weak he'll welcome the disaster.*

David found the voices uncannily clear, even though he suspected they came from inside himself. Later, when they talked again, he began writing down everything that was said. It became clear to him that the voices were discussing his eventual fate at the hands of homosexuals, who kept tempting him and thereby exposing him to scandal and professional ruin before his career had begun. By this time, curiously, he believed he had done something – as a cumulative effect of his little 'penances', perhaps – to write off the theft, and it no longer troubled him. The voices did trouble him, though, and after a few days he had accepted that they were real, and were saying things he should heed and act upon.

'They were not anything he imagined,' said Dr Loomis. 'He dismissed that idea very quickly. Now he *knew* they were real, and he didn't question their source. The important thing was, he was being privileged to overhear them and take warning from what they said. He was also managing to distance himself from any suggestion that he was homosexual – it was the others who were that way, not him, and they malignantly corrupted him by playing on what was no more than a weakness.'

David went about his business as outwardly cheerful as

ever, making customers smile, while the voices kept on talking, never addressing him directly, discussing his case and his chances of survival.

If he doesn't do something soon, one of them kept saying, *then there'll be no hope for him, he'll go down the black hole for good...*

Roughly ten days after the voices began, a man propositioned David in a coffee shop during his lunch break. David felt an immediate attraction, but the warning was just as immediate. He felt it and he heard it at the same time: *Now he has to do something...*

He spoke to the man, keeping him interested, and suggested they meet after work, at a place they both knew, a bar frequented by homosexuals. The man agreed, David returned to the bank and complained he was not feeling well. The manager told him to go home.

He took a taxi to a commercial district of the city where his face was not likely to be known. He went into a specialist cutler's showroom and told the assistant he wanted to buy a razor as a gift for his grandfather. He was shown a range of splendidly crafted instruments, and bought one with a mother-of-pearl handle. He also bought a strop.

At his assignation in the gay bar that night he deliberately kept to the shadows and was careful that no one other than his companion had a good look at his face. When the time came for them to move on, the man told David his car was out front. They got into it and the man drove to a remote spot, where he parked and switched off the engine.

'David took the initiative,' Dr Loomis said. 'He had planned this part of the evening meticulously, so he had to be in charge of the proceedings. A point arrived when the other man was exposed and in a state of some excitement. Holding him firmly with one hand, David drew out the razor with the other and removed half the man's penis in three or four strokes.'

David left the car at once, hearing the man screaming as he ran off down the road. When he got home he examined himself for signs of blood, but there were none. The razor rested in a plastic bag in his pocket with what he called 'reassuring weight'. Examining the instrument in the bathroom, he found only a tiny speck of blood dried on the side of the blade.

'I felt calmed by what I had done,' he told Dr Loomis. 'And the voices had stopped, they didn't start up again for days, and all during that time I felt calm and really very good. It was rationalised by then, see? I'd taken up arms against the enemy at long last, so obviously I would feel better, wouldn't I? I felt better because in a marginal way I really was a better person. The evil in me was their influence – it was *them*. They were the badness in my existence. If they went, my evil went.'

A week or so later David was propositioned again, and again he accepted, this time suggesting a children's play area in a park where homosexuals went at night. On this occasion he wasted no time on preliminaries. Less than five minutes after the man had made contact with David, he had slashed his genitals and run off.

'That case worried him to some extent,' Dr Loomis said. 'The first one made the papers, and the victim had claimed he was set upon by black youths who mutilated him and stole his wallet. The second man, however, never came to the notice of the authorities, even though David knew he had injured him really seriously. To this day he has never come forward.'

David's contact with reality grew weaker over the following

months. He tried to mutilate two more men, frightening the first one away before he could harm him, then cutting his own hand badly the second time. As he sat in an emergency department having the wound stitched, the voices started up again.

It isn't enough. He does what he can but it's not enough, it's not sacrifice enough. He is infested, he must know that. It's the infesting that will take him and drive him down the black hole. . .

The same words were repeated over and over, at intervals, for the next two days. During that time David also developed the delusion that a particular early-evening television programme was being directed at him, sending out coded bulletins about how well he was avoiding detection, and telling him what he must do if he wanted to stay free of the attention of the law and bad fortune in general.

'It had something to do with the Jack and the Beanstalk story,' David told Dr Loomis. 'I never quite picked it up, but I was to be sure that beans, or seeds, or roots about the house or garden, didn't harbour the makings of revealants – they were big creatures operating as force fields who could influence the airwaves around me and transmit my thoughts to the police. I cleaned out all the beans and seeds and other stuff I could and replaced them with harmless ones, but I was never sure if I was getting it right, or if the story was even Jack and the Beanstalk in the first place.'

Since starting to hear the voices and embarking on his campaign of mutilating homosexuals, David had been completely celibate. Dr Loomis believed that the consequent sexual tension, combined with the misgivings expressed by the voices, drove David to his next extreme act.

He went out one evening, telling his mother that he had arranged to meet friends at the squash courts in the sports centre. He went straight to a gay bar, picked up a young man and half an hour later had sex with him. On this occasion David made no attempt to mutilate his companion. Instead, he went to a lonely spot near a cemetery, where he slashed his own genitals and then sat waiting to be rescued or to die, whichever was decreed. He passed out from the pain and loss of blood and was found by a passing police patrol shortly before daybreak. In hospital it took a transfusion of five pints of blood and several hours in the operating theatre before a spokesman could tell his parents that he would survive.

Dr Loomis described the transformation that took place when David returned to consciousness.

'The first thing he told the nurses, as soon as he came round and could figure out what had happened, was that he didn't want to see his family, or anybody he had ever known before. It was over, he said, the old life was behind him, he was cleansed and his new existence meant all former connections had to be cut off – that was his choice of words.'

Although David expressed some disappointment that his genitals had been saved and he was still technically capable of sexual activity, he took comfort from the 'obvious fact' that this had happened so that he might go on being tested, in a minor way, so he wouldn't ever get the idea that being pure and staying away from the fleshly pursuits was entirely easy.

'To anyone encountering him and talking to him at that time, he appeared completely rational,' Dr Loomis said. 'He was able to analyse and dismantle his earlier motives and drives, and he could put up some pretty convincing arguments for the wrong decisions and bad turnings he took. But as time passed the reality began to submerge,

and although he still talked intelligently and thoughtfully
and with some very mature insight, he was now talking
about motives, drives, decisions and wrong turnings that
had never happened. He got himself an alternative past life
right out of the blue, with just enough real details in it to
appease his remaining traces of clear memory.

'All in all, if you didn't know anything about him, he
would have come across like a very bright guy just spending
some post-operative time in hospital, rather than a dangerous psychotic with no compunction about mutilating other
human beings at the prompting of imaginary voices.'

While police tried to question him about his victims and
piece together the pattern of his activity in the weeks and
months leading up to his self-mutilation, David began to
sink into inactivity. He communicated very little, and
appeared to be entering a chronic phase of his illness, which
had already been diagnosed as Paranoid Schizophrenia.

After four weeks of being relatively passive, he suddenly
leapt out of bed one morning and demanded to see
'Andron'. When he was asked who that was, he said he
could tell when people were lying, and if they didn't want
to help him he would help himself. Andron was in the
hospital, he said, and he had to locate him. Eventually
David was calmed and persuaded to take a tranquilliser.
When he was relatively settled Dr Loomis came to see him.
He asked who Andron was, and why the urgent need to
find him.

'I'll know him when I see him,' David said, 'but until I
see him I don't know what he looks like or who he really
is. All I know is if I don't make contact with him I'll slip
down and I'll never get up. I'll suffocate in the silt of dead
brain cells. This place is full of them.'

In spite of sedation David remained restless, insisting

over and over that he must see Andron. He hit a male nurse who tried to straighten his bedding and told him that if he didn't keep his disgusting hands to himself he would be reported to the 'chief technician' for his filthiness.

At some point between one nurse taking a break and another covering for him, David got out of his room at the hospital and went in search of Andron. He entered every ward, managing to stay beyond the reach of everyone who tried to catch him, and when he had been everywhere and looked at everyone in the hospital – including two dead men in the mortuary – he went to the kitchen, armed himself with a cleaver, and demanded to speak to Dr Loomis. It took an hour to locate the psychiatrist, but when he arrived David was still in the kitchen, still wielding the cleaver.

'Andron's left here,' he told Dr Loomis. 'Do you know what that means?'

'No. Tell me.'

'I have to bring him back. We have to make contact, you see. He doesn't know that, but he will when it happens, it'll be all right. But I've got to get him back here as soon as I can. You'll have to tell Loni. She can make him come.'

Dr Loomis suggested that David put down the cleaver, then they could make arrangements for Loni – David's girlfriend – to come in and get underway with the search. But David shook his head. He would make no deals or concessions.

'Bring her here and I'll talk to her. Tell her it has to be fast. The white count is going down.'

Loni did not want to go. David's secret life was no longer a secret to her and she did not think she could face him. Dr Loomis argued, gently, that a few minutes of her time might defuse a dangerous situation that could become disastrous. As if that were a cue, Dr Loomis' beeper went off a few moments later and he went to the telephone. His office patched him through to the hospital, where he was told that David had just killed one of the kitchen staff. The man had tried to make it to the exit door past David, who had leapt up, screamed at the man to get back, then began chopping at his head and neck with the cleaver. When the man was dead David settled down again and was back at his position in the middle of the kitchen, wielding the cleaver and demanding to speak to Loni.

She eventually agreed to go to the hospital when the local police chief promised she would be fully covered by his men when she spoke to David. When she arrived and was led to the door of the kitchen, David did not recognise her – she had changed the style and colour of her hair. Having gone that far to accommodate the authorities, Loni now made a serious effort to win David's confidence; as she spoke to him from the doorway he recognised her voice, and finally accepted that she was indeed Loni.

He told her to come in, he had to speak to her privately. Again the police chief reassured Loni she was being covered. She went into the kitchen. She had to walk round the body of the dead man to get to where David was standing.

'You have to take the essence,' he said, smiling at her.

Loni told him she didn't understand. Wasn't she to find Andron?

'That was a decoy ploy,' he said. 'Take the essence out with you. Put it on the stairs, it'll get lifted.' Then he nodded at her hand. 'Leave your finger, so you'll come back.'

Loni lost her nerve and as her expression changed and she stepped back, David grabbed her and swung the side of the cleaver against the side of her head. She fell and he raised the cleaver over her with both hands. At that moment a police officer shot him twice through the heart. Loni scrambled to her feet and was at the kitchen door before David's body had dropped to the floor.

'If the case taught me anything,' Dr Loomis said later, 'it's that I know practically nothing about the disorders of the human mind. I'm feeling my way in the dark with a few small reliable rules throwing their feeble light into my ignorance. Up until the moment David hit Loni I saw it all unfolding – he would talk with her, there would be appeasement, we would get him out of there and therapy would eventually do some kind of mending job on him. How wrong could I be? He wanted to mutilate her at the very least, and at the finish he was going to kill her. So I was reminded of the scope of my ignorance, that was my total gain from that case.'

There was also, he added, the reminder which could never crop up often enough: Paranoid Schizophrenia is potentially the most dangerous psychiatric illness of them all.

10
Sadomasochism

Sadism takes its name from the Marquis de Sade, who wrote stories about people who derived sexual pleasure from torturing helpless victims. Sadism, therefore, is defined as a form of sexual perversion characterised by the enjoyment of inflicting pain or suffering on others. Freud's view was that sadists could fend off the fear of castration and attain sexual pleasure only when they were able to do to another person what they feared might be done to them.

Masochism is named after Leopold von Sacher-Masoch, an Austrian novelist whose books, notably *Das Vermächtnis Kains* (The Legacy of Cain) and *Falscher Hemilion* (False Ermine) depict the abnormality of sexual gratification derived from one's own pain or humiliation. Analysing this perversion, Freud said that the ability of masochists to achieve orgasm is disturbed by feelings of sexual guilt which are eased by their own suffering.

A sadomasochist has elements of both sadism and masochism in his personality, and his sexual activities tend to be governed by one or the other. Since Sadomasochism is the joining of perversions which are respectively concerned with dominance and submission, it is therefore an exaggeration of conventional sexual activity between men and women. Society still expects that the male should take the lead (or aggressive) role in any sexual activity. The distinguished psychiatrist Anthony Storr has pointed out that the formation of the genitals demands that the male should thrust and penetrate, while the woman, even though she can be very mobile, is obliged nevertheless to be receptive.

In the book *Sexual Behaviour in the Human Female*, Kinsey and his fellow researchers point out that the human body, when subjected to functional analysis, displays a close link between sexual arousal and aggression. They provide a list of fourteen body changes which are common to sexual excitement and anger, and show that there are only four detectable differences between one state and the other.

The psycho-analytic explanations for Sadism and Masochism are not very satisfactory. Dozens of theories have been put forward, but the views which hold sway suggest that Sadism is rooted in the balance of loving and aggressive feelings the child experiences in the early relationships with its parents; the predominant theory about Masochism says that, because it is Sadism turned inwards, it can be explained in the same terms as Sadism.

In many cases of murder there are clear signs of sadistic motivation. The 'Monster of Düsseldorf', Peter Kürten, experienced orgasm when he stabbed or choked his victims. John Christie, who killed seven women, masturbated over their bodies or had intercourse with them after they had died.

'People who engage in sexual bondage and perform little sadistic rituals – often they're married couples – are on a different and much friendlier planet than the types who act on their impulses with no regard for the feelings of the other person,' said Dr Brent, a forensic psychiatrist from New York. 'I'm aware some of these people who indulge in sadomasochism for recreation have a tendency to believe there's something wrong with their heads. A lot of them come looking for help. But the real bad guys, the pathological cases whose pleasure comes at the price of human pain or misery and sometimes death, don't want any help. They want to stay the way they are, and if they ever come to our attention it's usually because somebody else complained about them.'

Brent believes that sadists and sadomasochists come from backgrounds where there has been very little love, and where they have learned from direct experience that prices have to be paid for every kind of advancement or pleasure.

'They don't identify with other people,' he said, 'because other people are alien. They do not see themselves as a part of any group, far less a society. They are solo, on their own, in confrontation with beings with whom they have nothing they want to share.'

The current trend of treatment for most sexual offenders is towards long-term group psychotherapy. This is opposed by large sectors of the public, and by certain elements within the psychiatric profession. Dr Brent believes that precious therapeutic time should be spent on patients with conditions which respond more positively to care and human contact. While he accepts that sexual offenders are people who have often been deliberately damaged, it does not follow, he says, that there is some onus on psychiatry or anybody else to go through the motions of trying to undo what probably can't be undone anyway.

'Sexual offenders, in my experience, have a group tendency to lie about everything, so when they seem to be responding to treatment, they most times are not. So the big flaw with a lot of the statistics is that they're based on the questionnaires which have been handed out to these liars. Sex offenders are like junkies, they'll say anything to get off the hook, or to get another fix, or to get the spotlight away from them. You may think I'm over-simplifying, but I'm not, I'm cutting across the crap and highlighting the hard facts. One such hard fact is this: psychotherapy for sex offenders is a waste of resources. From wide experience I can say that the sexual drive does not seem very amenable to psychological maintenance and repair. Usually I put it another way – a man who is led by his dick doesn't respond well when you treat his head.'

CASE ONE: *A Respectable Man*

Paul was a thirty-two-year-old Dutch television producer who found himself being plagued by progressively stronger sadistic impulses. He had been married for twelve years and for the past five years or more, he had had sexual intercourse with his wife on average twice a month. Since childhood, however, his sexual fantasies had been predominantly homosexual. He did not respond to his homosexual impulses in an overt way until after he was married, and even then, for a considerable time, his indulgence was relatively passive; he would spectate at live male sex shows in Amsterdam, and he bought large quantities of homosexual pornography, much of it with a sadomasochistic content.

'I was never drawn as strongly to heterosexual pornography as I was to the homosexual stuff,' he told a forensic psychiatrist. 'And the sadism and masochism in the hetero magazines did nothing for me.'

He had married for reasons of propriety, believing that

his future as a stable married man would be important to the advancement both of his career and his standing in the community. He also hoped that a regular heterosexual relationship would cure him of his homosexual tendencies.

'It didn't work, of course. I think I got worse, because I felt cut off from choice. I always thought of a man when I had sex with my wife, and I had a lot of homosexual masturbation fantasies, most of them involving bondage and beatings, sometimes featuring well-known men. I worked on a programme with a couple of film actors once, and both of them at different times had already played prominent parts in my fantasies. It was eerie.'

In his late twenties he began to frequent gay bars. He soon learned that the 'S & M' (sadomasochist) crowd had their own specific haunts. They wore clothes which signalled their preferences and appeared to communicate in numerous coded ways, using open, unambiguous, two-way speech only as a last resort.

'I resisted these people for a long time. Part of me, some bourgeois streak, rejected them quite firmly. I could see what was squalid about them, what was weak and despicable. For a while I could let my revulsion outweigh my fascination and curiosity. Then one day, I don't know, I'd had a bad few hours at the studios, I was angry and frustrated, nothing had worked out right, and on an impulse I walked out of the office, got in a cab and had the driver drop me off in the district where all those bars are clustered. I went into one, sat at a table near the bar, not being too blatant, but not making myself exactly withdrawn, either. Eventually I was approached.'

The man who spoke to him was circumspect. He asked if he might join Paul, and for a time he talked lightly and fleetingly about politics, the weather, the hopeless traffic situation, and then quite abruptly – perhaps sensing Paul's genuine nervousness, and his readiness for a new experience – he put his cards on the table. He told Paul he was sexually aroused by being beaten.

Paul had an impulse to leave ('My bourgeois streak again, I suppose . . .'), but he made himself stay, and he admitted he had never done anything active in the way of S & M. But the man reassured him, telling him he looked like a natural, keeping the tone half-joking as he said Paul was a real dominator if ever he saw one. They eventually went to the man's house where Paul beat him with a belt, being sure not to let himself go, taking care not to hit the man too savagely. Afterwards they returned to the bar and had a drink together. Paul had a feeling the man was slightly disappointed with the session.

'It was a strange experience, that first time,' Paul told the psychiatrist. 'I couldn't enjoy myself, it was all too new, and I felt awkward and fearful I might injure him. But afterwards, thinking about it, picturing the scenario and the trappings and the way he howled when the belt hit him, I got very aroused.'

He became so aroused, in fact, that he slipped back to the neighbourhood of the bar and was propositioned before he even got inside. This time the pick-up was strictly homosexual and the young man expected to be paid. Paul suggested a drink first, and thinking the situation through, he realised he was getting into something he had not planned and did not particularly want. He gave the young man money and left him there. That night he made love to his wife, picturing what had happened earlier with the man bound up and begging for mercy.

A week later he went to another S & M bar, appropriately dressed this time, so that his preference would be recognised. He was approached almost at once by a young man, probably eighteen or nineteen years old, who told Paul he had a place nearby. They had one drink, then left. At the apartment the youth explained the dramatic situation he liked, then let Paul strip him, bind him with straps and beat him with a whip. This time Paul was aware that he had not exercised so much self-control as before. Afterwards, the youth's lip was bleeding, and Paul was genuinely surprised to learn he had punched him.

'After that I visited the bars every ten days or so, and I learned to enjoy myself as much as my partners did. But I was always a shade concerned about the way I could let go now. Afterwards I couldn't always remember what had happened. Then one day I realised I had beaten a man unconscious. I panicked and ran away. For days I kept scouring the newspapers to see if I'd killed him. Thinking it over, I realised that it wasn't my awareness at the time that was faulty – it was my memory afterwards. What I did, however vicious, was controlled and deliberate. But at that time I did have a lot of fear about actions and their consequences. It faded, of course.'

A feature of dedicated sadomasochists is that they will develop a specific ritual framework of their own, which can become a trademark. Paul's was to tie up his partner – who always had to make a show of resistance – then taunt him with a knife, making the man whimper; a beating with a rope or a belt would follow, during which Paul would have an orgasm spontaneously, or if he did not, he would pretend to force his 'victim' to perform oral sex on him.

'It became an obsession with me,' Paul said. 'I could still work effectively, but only because I worked in educational broadcasting where my work was safe and undemanding. My mind certainly wasn't on what I was doing. Most of the

time I was fantasising about beating someone up, and in
the fantasies I would go much further than I did in real
life. Quite often I fantasised killing a man.'

About a year after he had begun going to the specialist
bars, Paul met a man who seemed to embody everything
he had been searching for. He was tall and strong looking,
fair-haired and Nordic, with facial features that reminded
Paul strongly of a boy he had worshipped at school.

'We were drawn to each other. I hadn't known him half
an hour before we were in his room, and in another five
minutes I was beating him, punching him mercilessly as he
rolled around in the straps, and when I began whipping
him I wanted to kill him . . . I wanted, specifically, to bring
about that erotic stillness of the dead, or certain dead men,
as I had imagined they would look, after dying from an
outpouring of violence . . .'

On that occasion Paul frightened himself badly. He
noticed, after his senses returned to normal, that his partner
was panting, obviously in some pain, and he was unable to
get himself out of the straps. Paul helped him and realised
he had a wound on his stomach.

'I had done it with the knife. I didn't know about it, not
until I saw it, and even then I don't remember doing it. It
was terrifying. I imagined killing somebody and not knowing I'd done it until the police came into my office and
grabbed me.'

Later, on an impulse, and still troubled by what had
happened with the fair-haired man, Paul went into one of
the bars pretending to be a masochist. In an encounter
which he could not remember well afterwards, he was
beaten so savagely that he had to drive himself to a hospital
and tell the casualty surgeon that he had been beaten up
in the street and robbed.

'Afterwards he tried to decide whether he had enjoyed the experience, savage and painful though the aftermath was,' the psychiatrist said. 'He decided he had liked it, but that he had no talent for picking out the kind of man who would not do him too much harm. He decided to stick to the aggressive role in future, not realising that his own partners had no way of telling, either, how violent he would be. It was something he didn't even know himself.'

At approximately this time Paul's wife found a bundle of his hidden pornography and confronted him with it. He tried to pass it off as research material for a documentary he was planning, but she did not believe him. She was obviously shocked at his preference. For a couple of years, she admitted, she had suspected he had been sleeping with his secretary, but she had said nothing because she did not want to disrupt the marriage. But she would not remain dormant or silent over a thing like this.

Paul managed to convince her it was all in his mind, a perverse little turn that he had always known was there and which he handled by looking at pornography and masturbating. His wife took it better than he expected: she said she supposed his effort to contain the problem and minimise it was a lot better than giving in to it and chasing other men.

He was so relieved by what she said – he hadn't wanted the marriage damaged, either – that he went out that same evening, telling her he was off to a rehearsal, and he picked up a slender youth and took him to a little hotel catering to the sadomasochistic fraternity.

'For the very first time in his life, this homosexual man had sexual intercourse with another male,' the psychiatrist said. 'It was more on the order of a rape, in fact. He felt such release, having brought even that fraction of his deviation into the marital light, that suppressed impulses were liberated. He had sex with the young man three times during the evening, then he tied him up, beat him, and had sex with him again before he took off the restraints.'

Paul now began to feel better about himself. He took a more direct interest in his work, he was more considerate to his wife, and his sexual drive intensified to a point where he was masturbating three or four times a day. He continued to pick up men and conduct fantasy scenarios with them. He regarded himself as more or less a fixed part of the Amsterdam S & M scene, as so many people seemed to be.

'Then he met Jeremy,' the psychiatrist said, 'and it seems the worst kind of chords were struck in both of them. Jeremy was totally submissive, but there was something about him that beseeched more and greater violence, and something in Paul responded, wanting to batter the life out of this weakling.'

That is what happened. At their third encounter Paul beat Jeremy senseless, raped him, then strangled him with a leather belt. He knew exactly what he was doing, and found he did not want to stop it happening.

'The actions were unrolling as if they had been rehearsed between us a thousand times,' he told the psychiatrist, 'I was in total control and he was the whimpering and shuddering instrument of my will, which absolutely *soared*, I had never known anything like that. When he died I knew he was going to die, and I gloated, I watched his eyes go dull and his tongue come out as his lips and cheeks turned purple. It was extraordinary, I was committing deliberate murder and it was the most enjoyable experience of my life.'

Paul wrapped the body in towels and the worn rug from the hotel room and threw it over the fire escape. He then left without being seen, went round behind the building and propped the body against the railings.

'It still went as if I'd rehearsed it to perfection,' he said. 'I brought round my car, bundled him into the boot, drove out to the brick kilns near Diemen and dropped him into the ash pit. It glowed red hot day and night, I'd heard about people disposing of all kinds of things out there, and I'd thought more than once that it would be just right for getting rid of a body. There was no one around, it was perfect.'

The psychiatrist noted that Paul felt no guilt over the murder, neither at the time nor in retrospect. When it happened he was elated, having done what he had fantasised many times. He could not make himself believe, even for a minute, that he would be caught for what he had done, or even suspected of it.

'The feeling of being impervious is typical of sadists, a fluctuating sense of immunity from all harm coupled to a sense of near-total control of their immediate destiny.'

For a time Paul's sexual drive seemed to calm. He compared it to the sated feeling after a rich meal. For a couple of weeks he did not feel inclined to go to an S & M bar, then one night, having sex with his wife, he fantasised killing again and experienced an orgasm of such violence his wife thought he was having a cardiac seizure.

'Next afternoon he was in one of the bars, looking for a collaborator,' the psychiatrist said. 'He found someone rather like Jeremy and rather rashly expected a re-run of things as they had happened before. But this man was difficult, he was reluctant, nervous, and after a while he didn't even seem to like Paul very much. That offended Paul deeply, since he was vain about his appearance and personality and believed he could prevail emotionally with any man.'

They drank and argued for a while, and finally, on the offer of money, the man agreed to go with Paul. They went to another of the seedy little local hotels where they could take a room by the hour.

The session did not go well. Paul could not get the echoes of the previous time out of his mind. He kept recalling the unstoppable surge of actions that culminated in Jeremy dying. The memory did not coincide very closely with the rather stilted action in the small room that day. He tried to think himself into the way things had been. This was a psychotic delusion he occasionally indulged in, a serious belief that he could influence events and even make circumstances, if not times, repeat themselves.

'It just got worse and worse,' Paul said. 'It wasn't my day, but I wouldn't accept that. Not now, not when I was such a unique entity, a *murderer* of all things! I must have placed a terrible strain on my psychic resources, because although I began to feel truly murderous, it was the kind of anger that has no power at its disposal. I was in a flat spin, when I should have been floating on air, bestriding the situation.'

In a final surge of impatience Paul hit the young man, knocking him semi-conscious, then laboriously raped him. He left the hotel before his partner had properly regained consciousness.

'Now there was an anger in him,' the psychiatrist said, 'a frustrated kind of rage that sustained itself on the memory of what he had done and had not yet been able to equal, or even approach. He was primed to bring about another death, he half-admitted it to himself. He wouldn't rest until he knew that he *could* do it again and experience that phenomenal sexual jolt. But this time, because of the anger, the impatience, and the wrong-headed belief that one experience can duplicate another – the event, when it happened, could not be under his control.'

The psychiatrist perhaps spoke with the certitude of hindsight, but he was correct. Paul eventually picked up another man, they went to the man's home and enacted a domination-submission scene. Paul had drunk more than usual and the alcohol sharpened his anger. It also made him very careless. He taunted the man with a knife, then cut him with it, on the shoulders and face. The man began to scream. Paul hit him with a strap, and when he would not stop screaming Paul stuck the knife into his chest. The man collapsed on the floor, with blood flowing freely from his wound and from his mouth.

Paul made no effort to cover his tracks. He left the house and was seen by several neighbours who had been alerted by the screaming. He drove to the television studios and went straight to his office. His secretary recalled that he was highly agitated and incoherent. He demanded to see all the recent correspondence on the current television series and began spreading it across his desk. Inevitably the police arrived a few minutes later. They asked Paul to account for his movements in the past hour and he denied he had been out of the building that afternoon. When the senior police officer suggested they continue the questioning at the station Paul sat down suddenly and said he would not utter another word until his lawyer was present.

Later that day Paul was charged with murder. He claimed he had suffered a brainstorm and had no recollection of the day's events. The forensic psychiatrist brought in to evaluate his state of mind said Paul's case appeared to be pretty typical of its kind. The only notable difference was that he was suddenly prepared to confess everything, so long as his testimony featured as part of a clinical interrogation, and not a police one.

'I'm so obviously a victim of my condition,' he said. 'I

imagine you'll be able to convince the court of that.'

At the trial the psychiatrist said Paul was cool-headed, calculating, and very intuitive about his own drives and motives. He was undoubtedly a man with a sexual disorder, but there was no fault in his sanity. He knew right from wrong and probably always did.

Under questioning by the defence, the psychiatrist agreed that, at odd times, Paul could have lost awareness of himself and what he was doing. 'But only,' the psychiatrist said, 'because he chose to let that happen. He knew about the possibilities of euphoria, and if the chance of losing control had ever troubled him, he was capable of disciplining himself to avoid anything like that ever happening.'

A jury found Paul guilty on two counts of murder. He was sent to prison for life.

CASE TWO: *Breach of Decency*

Louise Dunkhill was a housemaid who entered service with a Church of Scotland minister, a widower, in 1943, when she was seventeen. People who paid any attention to her said Louise was a plain, wholesome-looking girl, quiet and withdrawn, who went about her work diligently without drawing attention to herself. It was not until her accidental death ten years later, when she slipped crossing the road in Inverness and was hit by a car, that light was thrown on the real Louise Dunkhill. As a result of police findings at the manse near Balloch, two people committed suicide and a third tried but failed.

'I was asked to make an appraisal of the pathological aspects of the case,' said Ronald Cameron, a retired psychiatrist who practised in Edinburgh for thirty-five years, dealing mainly with patients classified as criminally insane. 'I was young and keen and anxious to make my name. In the circumstances I could have got myself a fine edge of notoriety, but at the time cases like this one couldn't be too widely publicised, because of the strictures surrounding breaches of public decency and so forth. Besides, certain people in the case had connections which touched the fringes of government in Scotland, so there was only a small local flap for a while, then all was silence.'

By the time Louise Dunkhill died at the age of twenty-seven, she had probably been involved in most perversions where a woman can actively participate. A trunk in her room at the manse was found to contain over 200 half-plate size photographs, immaculately hand-printed and sepia-toned to 'archival' permanency; most of the pictures featured Louise in fetishistic clothing, and all were obscene.

'There aren't many laughs in my business,' said Dr Cameron, 'but the thought of all that leather fetishism throbbing away under the bombazine surface up there at a Highland manse made me giggle. In picture after picture, Louise posed in leather corsets, thigh boots with incredibly high heels, shiny leather gloves that joined across her shoulders – all the paraphernalia, complete with whips and shackles. Her male slaves in the pictures were always sad or agonised looking, although their sexual excitement was never in doubt.

'The pictures covered the period from 1944 to roughly the time of Louise's death in 1953. You can see her assurance growing, the older she got. The dramatic expressions got better, she struck more voluptuous poses, she laid hands on her male companions with more obvious relish. We don't know the whole story, of course, but I didn't get the impression anybody had to coax Louise too hard to get involved in sadomasochism.'

Louise's co-conspirators were the minister and a local

lawyer called Duff, a first cousin of the minister. Duff was also identified, from the beginning of the investigation, as the person who had taken the photographs. Mr Duff's sepia-toning method, which used a conventional ferricyanide-bromide bath technique, but in unconventional proportions, gave his prints a rich coloration which was unmistakable, and was immediately recognised by a senior police officer, who was a member of the same photographic society as Mr Duff.

'They weren't simply a naughty-picture circle,' said Dr Cameron. 'In several of the pictures there were children, frightened-looking children, and three different young women, usually being abused in one obscene way or another by Louise or her companions. The pictures were certainly posed, and with a lot of care, but they were just as obviously intrusions into something not so formally organised, something quite dark and measurably dangerous.'

In one picture a trussed-up child, a boy of six or seven, was seen to be bleeding from the mouth; in another a little girl had weals across her shoulders; another showed a boy being sodomised by Louise using a leather phallus, and the child was in obvious pain.

Less that twenty-four hours after being confronted with the photographs the minister drank half a bottle of Lysol. He died within minutes, and in great pain. The lawyer, Mr Duff, did not seem to take such a tragic view of the discovery. He tried, in fact, to make it seem as if the whole thing was little more than a harmless lark that any red-blooded man would be glad to be caught up in.

'Who's to say what's right and normal,' he remarked. 'I can't say I was ever plagued much with guilt over what went on.'

He admitted that he had engaged in sadomasochistic

practices at the manse for a number of years, after being introduced to the 'leather capers' as he called them, by the minister in 1932, when they visited Germany together and the minister had taken Duff to a specialist brothel.

'The real activist in our revels,' Duff told the police, 'the one who had the most profound zest for what we got up to, was Louise. She took a deep, profound pleasure in causing pain, and it was sexual pleasure, open and blatant. I never agreed with that business of hurting children, but she engineered it all, she was the one who arranged the extra-curricular encounters.'

The police could not accept that Duff was as marginal a character in the case as he made out, but it became clear that Louise Dunkhill really had controlled the weekly orgies and fixed most of the rules. Duff said that his cousin, the minister, had involved a whole series of housemaids in his perversion over the years, but only Louise had taken to it wholeheartedly, eventually surpassing the minister in imagination and sheer nerve.

'She actually slaughtered a chicken one night, right there in the study with the rug rolled back and a groundsheet on the floor,' Duff said. 'She went through the ritual as if she had done it a hundred times before, yet it was the one and only time she ever did it, as far as I know. She stood there in her boots and nothing else, knife raised in one hand, chicken wriggling in the other. She swiped the knife across its neck and the head flew clean off, then she gripped the flapping body between her thighs until it stopped moving. The look on her face made me wish I could get half that much enjoyment out of anything, anything at all.'

Duff stubbornly denied that he knew the identity of the children in the photographs, and added that in any case they would now be much older and probably not recognisable from their pictures. The police made enlarged prints of the faces and had copies distributed to a number of police forces in the north of Scotland, but no identifications were ever made. One of the three young women featured in the pictures was identified by a police constable, however: she was a clerk employed by the Ministry of Food in Inverness.

'But she's in hospital just now,' the constable said. 'She tried to gas herself two or three days ago.'

News of the scandalous discoveries at the manse had travelled and the young woman had, on her own admission, 'panicked, I just lost my reason, I couldn't face the way things were turning out. I knew about the pictures, of course, I remembered them every time I saw Louise Dunkhill in the street. She always looked right through me, but I couldn't forget. Once I tried to talk to her, I wanted to ask her to burn the pictures, but she brushed me away as if I was attacking her. I was a very headstrong and immoral girl back in those days,' she added; 'I was wild, far too wild. I think I've paid for it, though . . .'

A few days after the police spoke to the young woman in hospital, the lawyer, Duff, got into a very hot bath in the early hours of the morning; sitting in the hot water he opened a vein in his arm with a razor. The heat drained his body of blood very quickly and he probably died within minutes.

'He suffered a great deal more than he let us think,' Dr Cameron said. 'The police found a long, rambling letter, too long to be called a suicide note, and in it he blamed himself for the fact that a private vice was having such public repercussions.'

> *... it was my idea that the photographs should be taken. If I hadn't talked Louise and my cousin into the idea, if I hadn't seduced them with my salacious arguments, then the death of Louise would have been no more than the closing of a tiny chapter, a simple passing with no reverberations. I am so sorry ...*

When the investigation was into its fifth week and the police, under various kinds of pressure, were on the verge of simply filing the case away, there was a third suicide. A teacher at a village primary school five miles from the manse hanged herself from a tree in her garden. She was Isobel Laing, an unmarried woman in her late twenties, reportedly a religious person who was highly regarded in the community. A police officer, seeing the body at the wayside mortuary, made the connection with the photographs found at the manse. Isobel Laing was one of the young women depicted in several 'torture' tableaux and a number of lesbian-domination poses with Louise Dunkhill.

'Over all, the case caused terrible pain,' Dr Cameron said, 'and I think I wound up feeling sorry for everybody involved. Among Louise's property in the trunk was a bundle of letters from the minister. It was odd, the passion he expressed for the dark princess, as he called her, and yet in their outward daily life – even, apparently, in their daylight dealings with each other – there was never a flicker of the powerful feelings they harboured.

'I think of that modest-faced, buttoned-up housemaid, moving among the rest of us with her darkness howling in her head and tearing at her body, and I can feel profoundly glad I'm too prosaic and unimaginative to qualify for that league of misery.'

11
Necrophilia

'This is the ultimate anti-life perversion,' said Dr George Kane. 'All of the sexual deviations, to some extent, deny the forward and upward nature of a healthy existence, but this one turns *everything* upside down, to the extent that the central object of sexual desire is a dead body.'

Sexual interference with the dead was known in ancient Egypt. Herodotus (484–425 BC) revealed in his massive *History* that when the wife of an important man died, her body was not given to the embalmers until three or four days had passed. This was a precaution to prevent the embalmers having intercourse with the corpse, which apparently happened often to the bodies of women who had just died.

E. Gregerson, in his book *Sexual Practices: the Study of Human Sexuality* (1983) describes a mock-copulation ceremony that was performed with mummies to restore a dead man's virility. The same author reports that at one time, the Indians of British Columbia allowed a man to show his grief by copulating with his dead wife. There is also evidence that until the eighteenth century, similar practices were common in Germany. Smith and Dimock, writing on Necrophilia in the book *Sexual Dynamics of Antisocial Behaviour* (1983), advanced the view that some of the most popular children's stories in the West have a strong necrophilic character – they cited 'Sleeping Beauty' as an example.

Necrophilia as a sexual preference is generally assumed to be uncommon, but some researchers have found it to be more widespread than might be suspected, and there never appears to have been a shortage of cases to study. A prominent authority was the German psychiatrist Krafft-Ebbing (1840–1902), who devoted the larger part of his career to forensic psychiatry and the study of sexual pathology. In his masterwork *Psychopathia Sexualis*, first published in 1876, he said that necrophiliacs could be divided into two groups: those who violate a body acquired when it is already dead, and those who first kill someone and then sexually abuse the corpse. In the latter case, according to another German authority, Hirschfeld, the violation of the corpse is triggered by a frenzy rooted in the aggressive and destructive impulse. 'The murderer is not satisfied by merely killing his victim,' he wrote, 'he also wants to possess her and destroy her beyond death.'

The case described here concerns a man in the second category of necrophiliacs.

CASE STUDY: *A Drama for Destiny*
Geoffrey lived in a rundown two-room apartment near Fort Hamilton, in the Bay Ridge area of Brooklyn, New York. In the summer of 1985 he was indicted for the murder of a nine-year-old girl. He did not deny the charge.

The court appointed a forensic psychiatrist, Dr Orville

Levi, to examine the prisoner and determine if he was legally sane at the time the crime was committed. Another forensic psychiatrist, Dr George Kane, quoted above, interviewed Geoffrey and investigated his history on behalf of the Prosecutor's Office.

'This was a twenty-eight-year-old unemployed man, rather shabby in appearance, with unkempt hair, a stubbly beard and clothes that were not particularly clean,' Dr Levi reported. 'On Sunday fourth August, the day of the crime, Geoffrey decided to spend the morning working on his toothpick model of St Patrick's Cathedral which, according to his wife, he had planned to sell for a lot of money when it was finished. Before he started he had two cups of coffee and three Quaaludes to steady his hand for the delicate work on the model . . .'

Quaalude is the trade name for methaqualone hydrochloride, a sedative drug with a barbiturate-like action. Because of extensive abuse this drug was eventually withdrawn from the market in the United States.

'He worked with the toothpicks and glue until about two o'clock,' Dr Levi continued, 'then he decided that because it was such a hot day, he would go downstairs and sit in the yard. His wife, who has a chronic drink problem, had already drunk half a bottle of rum that day and she had gone back to bed. When Geoffrey left the apartment he remembered to take his pet rat, which he was accustomed to carrying around with him, perched on his shoulder.'

As he sat on the ground at the rear of the building, playing with the rat, talking to it and letting it crawl from one hand to the other, he was aware that a small group of children were watching him. After a while, when he had let the rat creep into his shirt pocket to sleep, he lay back and closed his eyes, knowing that the children were still watching. One of them, the eventual victim, had attracted his interest.

'The minute I saw her,' he told Dr Levi, 'it occurred to me, this could be her, this could be the one who would take me into a new phase of my life.'

Later, as the children played around the edge of the yard, Geoffrey approached the little girl and took her aside. He asked her if she wanted to see the place where he made ice-cream. She was a trusting child who was not naturally suspicious of adults. She nodded enthusiastically. Geoffrey told her there wasn't enough ice-cream for everybody, so she was to wait until he had gone around the end of the building, then follow him as soon as the others weren't looking.

The girl did as he told her. When she joined him he led her to a derelict carpenter's yard a quarter of a mile from the apartment building. On the way he distracted her by letting her see the rat and stroke its nose. At the yard he led the girl to a dusty old hut and told her to look inside. The ice-cream, he said, was still churning round in a big tub right at the back.

'He stood behind her as she tiptoed into the hut,' Dr Levi said, 'and as she stepped into the shadows he made his decision. He was going to kill her. He went in behind her, grabbed her tightly round the neck and squeezed with both hands. The girl struggled, though not as hard as he had expected, and he kept on squeezing until he felt something in her throat give way.'

When Geoffrey let the girl go she dropped to the dirt floor. He knelt beside her. His whole body was shaking violently. He lifted her head and let it fall a couple of times, convincing himself she was dead. The third time he lifted her head her eyes fluttered open and she made a croaking sound. Panicking, he began punching her face, holding the back of her head with the other hand, feeling her facial bones crack under the impact of his knuckles.

'There was blood everywhere,' Geoffrey told Dr Levi. 'I couldn't believe there was so much of it. It all came out her mouth and her ears. I grabbed a couple of old paper sacks, cement bags I suppose, and I pushed her into one, just kept shoving her with one hand, holding the sack with the other, until she went inside. She was so light, it was incredible, she slipped in there like laundry. I folded over the top and pushed it inside the other bag. I put the bundle on a barrel beside the door and started kicking around the dirt and dust, getting rid of the blood. I guess I made a pretty good job, though I wasn't seeing too well. It was dark in there and I was getting strung out, all shaky, scared I'd get caught.'

When he had cleared the floor of traces of blood, he stood looking at the paper bundle on the barrel, feeling thwarted. The stress of finally having to punch the life out of the child had buckled his drive. He had been intent on having sex with the body, but now he knew he couldn't get an erection, he couldn't get himself lustful and avid in such a jumpy, half-shocked condition. He nearly cried, he said, standing there in the gloom, realising that if he didn't have sex with the dead girl then he would have killed her for nothing.

'It would have been a whole lot of strain and struggle for no payoff.'

He could not even bring himself to open the sacks again. Finally he stood them on the floor, turned the barrel upside down and slid it down over the bundle, hiding it completely. He shut the door of the hut and went home.

In the tiny kitchen he found his wife cooking herself an

omelette. She asked if he wanted one but he said no, he wasn't hungry, and blamed the heat for his uncharacteristic lack of appetite. He sat down at his model again and pretended to make adjustments to the frontage with a craft knife and a glue brush. When his wife finished eating her omelette she smoked a cigarette, then told Geoffrey she felt sick and needed to lie down. She went back to bed.

Geoffrey sat motionless in the apartment until it turned dark, testing his feelings over and over, trying to gauge how different he felt now that he was a murderer.

'In retrospect,' Dr Levi said, 'he believed he must have been in shock, because his mind seemed to go into a loop, travelling the same territory endlessly, rescreening the scene in the hut. At approximately midnight he took three more Quaaludes, because he felt he needed them, and shortly afterwards he decided he would go back and make sure the body had not been disturbed.

'He had a vague plan to move it to somewhere else, where he could keep it for his own use, but that was just a piece of flimflam, a reactive non-decision. He did that a lot, it was a habit, he conjured so-called schemes out of the air to delude himself – and other people – that he was a decisive kind of man with a direction in life.'

Before leaving the apartment Geoffrey put a candle and a packet of matches in his pocket. As he left the building he was approached by a tearful young woman who asked him accusingly if he had seen her daughter. Geoffrey told her gruffly that he didn't know what she was talking about, but a small boy shouted from an open doorway that he was the man his sister had gone away with. Geoffrey brazened his way out of the confrontation, insisting he hadn't been further than the back of the building all day. He sauntered off in the opposite direction to the yard where the body was hidden. Keeping his pace slow and casual, he made his way back by a circular route that added more than a mile to the trip.

In the hut he put the candle on the floor and lit it. The angle of the light and the dramatic long shadows in the cobwebbed interior fired his sense of drama. He removed the barrel from the nested sacks, opened them slowly and pulled out the girl's body.

'Her face looked black with the dried blood,' he said. 'Her hair was tangled and stuck in the cuts on her face. She looked terrible, really, but it suited the way things were. It was part of the drama. I laid her on the floor, straightened her out, then I stood and looked at her for a while.'

As he stood there staring, Geoffrey became sexually excited. He took the clothes off the body and managed partial penetration. In spite of the awkwardness and discomfort he reached orgasm and felt, finally, that it had all been worthwhile.

He put the corpse back in the sacks and covered them again with the barrel. At that point, he recalled, he was wondering how long he could keep coming back to have sex with the body, before it became too badly decomposed.

Walking home, he saw a knot of people outside his apartment block. As he drew nearer he could see a couple of police uniforms under the street lights. An officer stepped forward and asked Geoffrey to identify himself. It was the beginning of an interrogation that ended at dawn in the police station. Geoffrey denied any knowledge of the missing girl and was finally released, with the promise that the police would be in touch again. He went home. His wife had gone off to her job as a shelf-filler at a local supermarket. Geoffrey took three Quaaludes and went to bed.

He slept until early afternoon. 'When he awoke,' Dr Levi

said, 'he seems to have been in a very agitated condition. It was probably more of a physical reaction than a psychological one – dehydration from the drugs, low blood-sugar from lack of food and so on, but he was really jumpy and he was convinced that in daylight somebody would find the body.'

Geoffrey threw on his clothes, slipped out of the apartment and hurried along to the derelict yard. In the hut everything looked just as he had left it.

He had been inside the hut for less than a minute when two police officers came in. They had followed him, of course. According to their testimony Geoffrey simply looked at them, shrugged, and pointed to the barrel.

Although Dr Levi studied Geoffrey's background history alongside other data relevant to the crime, it was Dr Kane, for the prosecution, who made an exhaustive study of Geoffrey's past.

Dr Kane is a severe critic of the 'charitable purblind' in his profession who confuse degeneracy with sickness and try, as he sees it, to put a clinical label on every disgraceful impulse a pervert will surrender to. Dr Kane admitted that he could not separate his own feelings from the investigation of Geoffrey's social and sexual history. 'It hardened my belief that certain individuals are beyond the reach of any kind of civilised redemption.'

Dr Kane worked back from Geoffrey's assertion, in the early stages of interview, that he believed he was destined to have sex with a corpse. It was, Geoffrey said, a stage in his development, a segment of the 'drama' which he must act out in order to achieve his destiny. He could not remember how long he had believed that, but he did know that for a year before he finally murdered the little girl, he had been sure he would have to kill to obtain a body – stealing one would have lacked the drama necessary for the fulfilment of his destiny.

'He really believed all that destiny crap,' Dr Kane said. 'Like a lot of inadequates, he was sure he was a big-timer underneath, something very special, a guy who was likely to break through one day and dazzle the whole world. I've come across the syndrome so many times I was prompted to come up with a slogan – *There Are No Half-Measures with Half-Brains.*

'It's like the ones who believe in reincarnation. They're nerds most of them, social and intellectual midgets, but they're convinced that in a former life they were Napoleon or Cleopatra or Attila the Hun. Nobody who believes in reincarnation was ever anybody ordinary or inferior. Not until now, that is.'

The social welfare office in Queens, where Geoffrey grew up, kept an extensive record of his early years. He had been a bed-wetter until he was eleven or twelve. He had a poor attendance record at school and was apparently an unruly child with a notably cruel streak.

'He was vicious,' Dr Kane said, 'a little goon from the time he was old enough to put kerosene in his baby sister's milk. There's a social-worker's record of him making a neighbourhood kid eat dirt then wash it down with his own urine. But Geoffrey's special talent was with animals. He liked to catch a cat and swing it by its neck on the end of a rope. Or set fire to kittens, he did that a couple of times – kerosene again.

'On a single afternoon he trapped four dogs and tied their front legs behind their backs. It seems he got a kick out of watching them push themselves along on their chests. I asked him what he could remember about his feelings at that period, going around doing things like that, and all he could say was, "I knew I was being driven to do it, because my spiritual nature comes from the dark side." He often sees himself as something diabolical, something richly evil. I had to bite my tongue to keep from telling him he doesn't have the personality or the style for evil.'

When he was five Geoffrey was forced to perform oral sex on a teenage boy. During his own late teen years he had homosexual relations with several boys while conducting a heterosexual affair with a married woman. He believed that he had sex in one form or another, including masturbation, at least once a day every day from the age of fifteen until some time in his early twenties.

'He was also a pervert from an early age,' said Dr Kane, 'a die-cast degenerate. He had all the earmarks – a tendency to look for an underside to every sexual act, a wallowing in anything unclean or aesthetically repellent, and a pre-occupation with humiliation, his own and other people's.'

Before he was fifteen Geoffrey was already experimenting with unusual forms of sex using fetishistic objects, and devices such as artificial vaginas and painful genital restraints. One night when he was approximately nineteen, he was performing a sado-masochistic act with a prostitute in a brothel when a girl in the next cubicle suffered a heart attack after sniffing an 'amy', a capsule of amyl nitrite, a heart-stimulant sometimes used to heighten orgasm. The girl died almost at once.

One of the prostitutes told investigating police officers how Geoffrey had gone into the cubicle and looked at the dead girl for a long time. 'He stood there in his leather and metal,' Dr Kane said, 'staring at her, his eyes moving over the body as if it were crucially important that he remember every detail.'

It was at this time, Dr Kane believed, that Geoffrey got his fixation of having sex with a dead body.

'The Necrophilia would have surfaced in the fullness of time, one way or another, given his proclivities and instincts. But at that particular time and in those circumstances the onset must have been especially vivid.'

A month before his twenty-first birthday Geoffrey was arrested for savagely beating a prostitute. She revealed to the police that he had paid her to impersonate a dead woman, an act which turned out to be just one of a number of specialities she provided for sexual deviates. Wearing a shroud and very pale make-up, she lay in a coffin set on trestles in a darkened room, with candles burning on either side. She told the police that Geoffrey had followed the ritual along its usual lines by lifting her out of the coffin, laying her on the bed, then raising her shroud and having coitus with her while she continued to pretend she was dead.

'But then he went haywire,' Dr Kane said. 'He dragged her off the bed, threw her on the floor and, according to the woman, after kicking her around he tried to bite a chunk out of her breast.'

This last detail, Dr Kane believed, showed that Geoffrey was also drawn to the practice of Necrophagy, in which a corpse is first mutilated, then parts of it are eaten.

'It's all so negative that it argues for the obvious,' Dr Kane added. 'These people, they are completely subtractive, they make no positive mark on the world. They are the walking equivalencies of drought, famine, plague and cancer. I know it's fashionable nowadays for the psychiatric establishment to wring its hands and say, "poor guy, let's try to help him", whenever somebody does what a Geoffrey does. What I say is, if we don't get realistic with a programme of exclusion on these people, if we don't harden up our attitudes about what's good and what's plain lousy, we'll just sink deeper and deeper into sentimental permissiveness and diluted judgement. Then before you know it, Necrophilia and Paedophilia and all the other philias will be regarded as nothing more than individualistic expressions of sexuality, mere quirks, and as enlightened citizens it'll be our duty to accommodate them in our everyday lives.'

As the interviews continued, Geoffrey revealed that from the age of twenty onwards he had regular fantasies about stealing a woman's body, or of killing a woman, tearing off her clothes and then, in his own words, 'doing all kinds of things connected with mutilation and sex.'

Running parallel with Geoffrey's unconventional sexual drive had been a long-standing interest in the occult. He could quote Biblical passages about death and damnation, and had made a hobby of memorising the prophecies of Nostradamus.

'He believed a day would come when his dark potency would prevail, and he would exercise the power of life and death over everybody else,' Dr Kane said. 'There's an amazing carbon-copy quality about the fantasies of perverts. They compensate in their heads, but unlike other people they do it wildly, they abandon reality, they have to convince themselves they're ultra-special. In a way they're like those amateur conjurors, the guys pulling doves from their coat tails who think they're being cool and mysterious and have a terrific edge on the others, when all along they're mostly socially compromised dweebs who talk funny and don't fool anybody with their tricks. But at least the magicians are harmless.'

The Bible and Nostradamus seem to exert a particular

magnetism on disturbed individuals, Dr Kane said. 'The Book of Revelation is popular with all kinds of degenerates, because it talks about the ascendancy of beasts, it hints at the power of cabbalism and other occult hocus-pocus, and of course it's nice and ambiguous – emotionally deformed and dangerous characters like Geoffrey tend to love high-sounding ambiguity, to them it's a lot like profundity. The Book of Revelation has a lot to answer for. It gives the repulsive fancies of perverts a hint of black-clad respectability.'

Geoffrey married his wife on the strength of prophecy, he told Dr Kane. In a dream he had been arrested for having sex with a dead child, and a woman came to the police station and said something to the desk sergeant, pointing to Geoffrey all the time she talked. Although Geoffrey strained to listen he couldn't hear, but whatever she said about him, they let him go. Her face had stayed with him after he awoke, and three weeks later he saw her in the flesh, working as a waitress in a diner.

'She was ten years older than me, but I knew I had to marry her,' he said. 'It was a unit of my destiny. I had to do it.'

Over the years Geoffrey vacillated between believing he was destined to be a messiah, and being convinced he was a son of Lucifer. Eventually, he decided that because his instincts were so distinctly unchristian he must be a devil, but he remained convinced that the Christian Bible was his coded handbook.

'It works by opposites,' he explained. 'Where the Bible says "do this", then I don't. When it says "don't do this", that's the route I'll take.'

Dr Levi, in preparing his determination for the court, pointed out that Geoffrey had a history of uncontrollable

sexual urges which were far from normal, and that he was
in every regard a misfit and undoubtedly dangerous. His
case history, taken overall, indicated that he suffered from
a serious personality disorder which had produced in him
the compulsion to kill.

'The personality disorder in itself does not justify a
defence of insanity,' Dr Levi told the court. 'The fact that
the defendant is also a necrophiliac, although horrifying to
contemplate, is no basis for an insanity defence, either. I
must conclude that at the time he committed the offence
with which he is charged and which he admits, he was
capable of realising his actions were wrong.'

Dr Kane's report agreed with that, adding that Geoffrey
was not suitable material for rehabilitation, since no
adequate treatment for Necrophilia had as yet been formu-
lated. Geoffrey was eventually sentenced to life
imprisonment.

12
Paedophilia

The word paedophilia literally means 'love of children'. In psychiatric classification, Paedophilia is a perversion characterised by an adult having a strong desire for sexual contact with children. The majority of paedophiles are male and they are mostly heterosexual, many of them being sexually inadequate in one way or another.

There are no reliable figures for the prevalence of Paedophilia, although from the extensive trade in child prostitutes in the East (catering mainly to visitors from the West) and the huge quantities of child pornography permanently circulating in Europe, it would seem that an interest in sex involving children is widespread.

Psychiatry puts paedophiles into two categories, Primary and Secondary. Usually, Secondary Paedophilia is an off-shoot of some other condition not related to Paedophilia, such as degenerative brain disease, a disintegrating person-ality condition or a genetic disorder. Sufferers in this cate-gory rarely appear before the courts and so are not often seen by forensic psychiatrists.

Primary Paedophiles, on the other hand, are regularly prosecuted under the criminal law – though certain authorities say not often or severely enough. This group is subdivided into two types, labelled Invariant and Pseudoneurotic. Some psychiatrists use the alternative terms 'fixated' and 'regressed'.

The Invariant (or Fixated) Paedophile is a man who has always been involved with children and adolescents; he has no sexual interest in adults. Frequently he has a shallow personality of limited range, with no special interests or enthusiasms, and he tends to live a solitary life. He shows no signs of guilt or shame about being a paedophile.

A Pseudoneurotic (or Regressed) Paedophile usually has an adult heterosexual relationship which doesn't run a particularly smooth course and is troubled from time to time by impotence, or some other inadequacy like premature ejaculation, which appears to be neurotic in origin and seems to distress him. At odd times, seemingly in response to overburdening stress, he commits a sexual act with a child. Afterwards he expresses a lot of guilt and shame. However, psychiatric studies of such men usually reveal that their lives are dominated by a sexual attraction to children which exists *at all times* under a veneer of conventional sexuality. Their potency in the adult sexual relationship often relies on paedophile fantasies entertained during sexual intercourse.

Worldwide research, particularly intense during the past twenty years, has produced statistics which give some idea of the 'average' paedophile, although there are, as usual, disagreements which tend to blur the picture.

Most studies find that the mean age of paedophiles at the time of arrest is mid-thirties; the age range is between seventeen and seventy. Strictly speaking this only tells us the age at which certain paedophiles get arrested, but some deductions can be made. For example, to puncture one myth, paedophiles are not mainly old men. It can also be argued that the numbers being arrested give a good idea of paedophilic activity at certain ages, which in turn throws light on the strength of the urge at different ages.

Basic sexual preferences are clear from all the studies – heterosexual paedophiles greatly outnumber homosexual or bisexual paedophiles. Most paedophiles over the age of twenty are married or have been married. Many of them practise other sexual deviations besides Paedophilia, e.g. Exhibitionism, Sadism, even Necrophilia. There seems to be nothing specific either in intelligence or education that would distinguish the paedophile from the rest of the population, although one researcher said she found the IQ of her paedophile subjects 'rather low'.

Studies designed to determine occupation and social class among paedophiles tend to contradict each other. One group of researchers reported that more than eighty per cent of subjects had skilled or semi-skilled jobs; in another study, the comparable figure was lower than forty-five per cent. A study of the paedophile self-help group PIE (Paedophile Information Exchange) showed that thirty-eight per cent were professional men, thirty-five per cent were white-collar workers, and fourteen per cent blue-collar workers. It has been argued that this statistic gives a warped picture of the average paedophile, since PIE was designed to attract articulate and well-educated individuals. Most studies do agree, however, that the majority of paedophiles grow up in conventional, stable families.

Many paedophiles claim that they are, to quote E. Brongersma in the *International Journal of Law and Psychiatry*, 'people who love children and want to express their feelings with bodily tenderness'. Another partisan argument is that Paedophilia was practised in ancient Greece and in other great civilisations down through the centuries.

'If that were the whole story it would be sound reason to write off the ancient Greeks as reprehensible and morally disgusting,' said a Canadian forensic psychiatrist, an authority on Paedophilia. 'But as so often happens with pleading on the part of criminals and perverts, the facts have been trimmed to suit their case.'

He cited a book by H. Licht, *Sexual Life in Ancient Greece*, which points out that sexual intercourse with boys or girls below the age of puberty was severely punished in ancient Greece, usually by flogging and sometimes by death.

A few professionals have tried to show paedophiles in a kindly, beneficent light (notably G. D. Wilson and D. N. Cox in the *British Journal of Hospital Medicine* in 1983), but hard evidence is stacked against them: paedophiles do serious harm to children. There are countless reports of anal and vaginal injuries, bodily bruising, cigarette burns, cuts, weals, bruises – all inflicted by paedophiles practising violence, much of it sadistic, against children.

'Even on the occasions when there is no sexual interference,' said the Canadian practitioner, 'a child's path to maturity is harmed by contact with adult sexuality. Anna Freud and others have made the observation and they've done the groundwork to prove it – if you involve a child in sexual practices for which he or she isn't yet ready, if you force the libido into premature flowering, then that child's development will be damaged.'

Group treatment and behaviour therapy have both been tried with paedophiles, but there is no convincing evidence that these produce good results. 'For the present,' said one therapist, 'we are dealing with incurables. A lot of the trouble lies in the fact that very few paedophiles want to be cured. In spite of occasional hardships, they like being the way they are.'

The causes of Paedophilia are not known. A number of theories are examined in Mohr, Turner and Jerry's *Paedophilia and Exhibitionism* (1964), and many papers on the subject have been published in Europe and America, all offering possibilities but none with enough evidence to draw a hard conclusion. If no clear causes emerge, a few chilling certainties do, and two of them are kept firmly to the fore when forensic psychiatrists make their evaluations:

All paedophiles are dangerous.

The younger his victim, the more dangerous the paedophile.

CASE ONE: *Born That Way*

Dr Pietro Marinetti was thirty-seven, unmarried, a successful paediatrician from Rome who took up a consultancy in Paris in March 1992. Marinetti's particular area of knowledge was child development from birth to the fifth year, and specific diseases associated with that period of life. He had written a book on his speciality, and because he was multilingual he was able to lecture widely across Europe.

In May 1993 Dr Marinetti was arrested and charged with gross indecency. Specifically, he was accused of fondling a number of boys from the area of Paris where he lived; the ages of the boys ranged from seven to thirteen.

Marinetti's colleagues were astonished. His friends simply couldn't believe it. Here was a man who devoted his life to the care and wellbeing of children, locked up in a cell accused of sexually abusing little boys. How could it be? His mother in Rome, learning of his arrest, suffered a near-fatal heart attack.

A forensic psychiatrist was engaged to make a pre-sentencing assessment. He learned that Pietro Marinetti's family background had been eminently stable and respectable. His father was a diplomat, a man who lived for his work and spent very little time with his four children. The mother on the other hand was attentive, loving and even-handed in the way she shared her time and affection with the children. Pietro had grown to be a studious and methodical young man, self-assured on the outside, with a clear determination to make medicine his career.

'I never had any doubt about my ability to get on,' he told the psychiatrist. 'I was a swot, I suppose, and I had a talent for categorising information inside my head. Intellectually I was robust and as self-assured as anybody could be. But I did feel unsure of my footing in the emotional world. I was out of step. From the age of five or so, I always wanted the company of boys.'

He had never experienced sexual attraction towards girls or women, and never towards adult males, either. As a child he had formed a powerful attachment to another boy and had experienced 'real heartbreak' when the boy moved away with his family to another town when Pietro was eleven.

'As time passed I got over him, but I noticed that as I grew older, my performance remained fixed. I was drawn most strongly to boys between eight and twelve years old. By the time I was sixteen I still sought out their company. I was always friendly and loving, I never harmed any of them . . .'

He would fondle the boys, arousing them, and encourage them to masturbate him. As he grew older this behaviour continued, and even as a junior doctor he would make advances to young patients in the paediatric wards.

'It was dangerous of course, from a professional and ethical point of view,' he said. 'But I never felt any *guilt*. Such feelings never seemed appropriate. No child was ever distressed by what I did, or by what I got them to do for me.'

Pietro's first sexual experience was at the age of seven, when a sixteen-year-old cousin from Turin sucked his penis on several occasions during a holiday visit.

'I never forgot the sensation. Soothing, like falling asleep, a dreamy kind of pleasure. I thought about it many times in the years afterwards, although my cousin never approached me in a sexual way ever again. Sometimes still when I dream I am there again, in my little bed, and he is bent over me, his head rising and falling gently as if he were grazing. But in the dream I am a grown man, and his attentions produce an orgasm.'

Paedophiles commonly minimise their perversion and claim it does no harm to the victims. Sometimes the paedophile will genuinely believe his distortions. The forensic psychiatrist who assessed Dr Marinetti was convinced he genuinely believed he did no damage to children.

'By stages over the years,' the psychiatrist reported, 'Marinetti had built up a defence which not only plays down the harmful psychosexual consequences of his games with children, but actually makes a case for the beneficial effects of paedophilic interference.'

Early arousal of the sexual instinct, according to the doctor's argument, is as beneficial to the child as an early acquaintance with reading and writing. 'It's been shown that a child who begins to learn early in life is capable of absorbing much more than one who starts late,' he said. 'Children who are able to acknowledge their sexual nature, and to indulge in the pleasures of sex, grow into adults with a greater capacity for the mature life. They arrive in adulthood with nothing fundamental to learn, so they spend their early adult years simply refining their sexuality, in the same way that they consolidate their intellectual gifts.'

So what about the ones who grow up to be paedophiles? he was asked. Didn't something in childhood, some sexual interference perhaps, slant their sexuality and distort it to the extent that they could not relate sexually to other adults?

'Not at all,' Dr Marinetti said. 'Certain children are destined to grow into the lovers of children. Paedophiles are born the way they are. There is no question of someone who is not orientated towards Paedophilia being *turned* that way. That's a myth which suggests that Paedophilia is a distortion of nature, and it has been put about by the disapprovers. People who are born with the same sexual orientation as myself have pleasant, relatively calm childhoods. The transition to adulthood is easier for us than for most others.'

Marinetti's own passage from boyhood into the adult state, however, had hardly been smooth. In his mid-teen years he continually fantasised about boys between the ages of eight and twelve. Whenever he masturbated, which was sometimes three times a day, he would always picture a boy in that age range, usually one to whom he felt some special attraction at that time. On his own admission he was frequently miserable and once or twice suicidal, when a boy failed to return his affection. For a time he assumed he would grow into an adult homosexual. It was only when he was nineteen or twenty that he realised his sexual drive was exclusively towards young boys.

'I did try to transfer my affections to women,' he told

the psychiatrist. 'From the point of view of professional stability it is always an advantage to have a wife.'

His efforts were disastrous. He could only bring himself to make advances to women who looked distinctly boyish, and of three he approached over a period of eighteen months, two turned out to be lesbians.

'The third one did respond to me, and when the time came I tried to have intercourse with her, closing my eyes and pretending she was a boy. But it was no good, I was impotent, and when she tried to arouse me with her hand I was almost physically sick.'

The forensic psychiatrist told the court that Dr Marinetti was a confirmed paedophile who could not believe that he was perverted, or that he was in any way a probable source of harm to young boys.

'His kindly intentions towards his sexual targets are probably genuine,' the psychiatrist concluded, 'and he has never used physical force to obtain sexual gratification. He remains, nevertheless, a potentially dangerous individual. He will agree to accept therapy, should the court decide his case merits such a course, although he does not believe he is in need of treatment of any kind.'

The psychiatrist was obliged to add that the failure rate of treatment for paedophiles who prefer children of their own sex is roughly double that of those who are drawn to the opposite sex.

The court made no recommendation about treatment. Dr Marinetti was sentenced to five years' imprisonment. He had been in prison ten weeks when a group of other prisoners attacked him. They dragged him from the refectory to the kitchens and held his head under a tap of near-boiling water. Marinetti suffered deep-level burning, lost all his hair and in time required extensive skin grafts. Eleven months into his sentence, he swallowed three razor blades and died of a massive internal haemorrhage.

CASE TWO: *A Mother's Warnings*

At Shellyville, Indiana, in the American Midwest, thirty-six-year-old Jan Gorter was arrested for molesting pre-pubescent girls. While awaiting trial he asked to speak to a 'sex expert' and was visited by Dr Martin Jonas, a forensic psychiatrist and university lecturer in abnormal psychology at Indianapolis.

'Jan Gorter had been brought up in a semi-rural community near Muncie, by lower-middle-class, first-generation Dutch immigrant parents who were not particularly well educated,' Jonas reported. 'The mother in particular was a staunch member of the NHK, the Dutch Reformed Church, and was considered to be severely prudish even by Dutch rural standards. She was the main influence on Jan during his boyhood, making sure he never got educated above his station. She filled his head with everything she felt he needed to know in order to lead a virtuous Christian life. It was bound to happen that her dominance in his youth had formidable reverberations in his later life.'

At the time of puberty Jan's mother deliberately frightened him with sexual myths and insanely exaggerated warnings about the hazards of enjoying himself. She told him that all women, from puberty up to the age of thirty, carried the germs of venereal disease. She explained that if he ever contracted syphilis – 'the worst and most terrible of all God's punishments' – it would attack his brain, making him first blind, then screaming mad.

'And she made sure he didn't turn to the solace of masturbation,' Jonas said. 'She told him that it was the vilest sin for a human being to touch his own genitalia for the purpose of inducing pleasure. She used the language of the Church, calling it "self-pollution", and warned the boy that his private parts would turn ulcerous and foul, and would eventually drop off if he ever abused them.'

Most damaging of all, Dr Jonas felt, was the mother's warning that any kind of sexual activity between adult men and women was evil and fraught with hazards so horrible they could scarcely be imagined.

'Jan wanted to question that, but he was trained to be obedient to his mother, and conditioned never to argue with her. Even though the stunted pathways of his own logic saw a flaw in her condemnation of human sex, he could not believe, deep down, that she was telling him anything but the awful truth.'

Jan had begun masturbating at the age of fourteen, a few months before his mother descended on him with her warnings; he stopped masturbating almost at once and suffered terrible feelings of guilt about his attraction to the opposite sex. As he grew older he became afraid of girls, yet he was still sexually drawn to them.

'I believed it was God's way of testing me,' he told Dr Jonas.

Since before puberty, Jan had been sexually aroused by watching the sexual activity of animals, and prior to abandoning 'self-pollution' he had used an image of a stallion and a mare copulating as an erotic fantasy. At school he had heard boys tell stories of human beings having sexual contact with farm animals, and in his physical-mental turmoil he began, at the age of fifteen, to have sexual intercourse with cows.

'As perversions go, bestiality isn't very common,' Jonas said. 'The underlying reasons in Jan's case were pretty unusual, too. But there was nothing half-hearted about his swing towards animals. He had coitus with cows practically every day between the ages of fifteen and nineteen.'

It took an outbreak of milk fever in local herds to put a stop to Jan's sexual activity. He associated the disease with syphilis, which terrified him.

'So now he was in a quandary,' Jonas said. 'He tried contact with other animals – sheep, a goat, even a dog, but they lacked the passivity of the cows and could turn very aggressive. It's a bizarre and frankly farcical scenario, but for him it was close to tragedy. What could he do? He was almost twenty and thanks to his mother's tampering with his psyche he was sexually overheated most of the time – *and* he was just as scared of grown-up women as he was of masturbation. It was a painful dilemma. It did not last long, however.'

Jan devised a compromise which he believed satisfied his taboos *and* his mother's version of Divine Justice, which she had assured him was eternally poised over his head like a cleaver.

'Coitus with young girls was forbidden, of course,' Dr Jonas said, outlining Jan's reasoning. 'He didn't like the idea of that anyway. But nevertheless, it was only sex between grown-ups that was evil, which in Jan's mind meant that sex between grown-ups and children was relatively OK. There was no danger of venereal disease, either, since only the big girls carried that particular plague. So Jan simply reverted to his pre-pubertic sexual-outlook, which was idyllic, since it predated his mother's hellish warnings.'

So, with a relatively clear conscience, Jan set out to cultivate the company of girls between the ages of ten and twelve, and found he had a talent for winning their confidence. In addition to fondling them sexually, he was usually able to persuade them to masturbate him – which was not wrong, since his mother had specifically said that the touching of *one's own* genitals was what constituted a sin.

Jan's sexual career with young girls lasted more than fifteen years before he was caught. Dr Jonas's diagnosis, appended to his report on his interviews with Jan, was Severe Paedophilia with a history of Zooerasty (sexual intercourse with animals). The court sent Jan to prison for five years.

While he was in prison he underwent behavioural therapy aimed at removing some of his taboos and directing his sexual energies along more acceptable channels. Part of the treatment was called Masturbatory Satiation: this required him to masturbate repeatedly, which he was eventually able to do, and to fill his head with erotic images of young girls as he did so. He was also given medication, cyproterone acetate (trade name Androcur), to lower his levels of testosterone, and, consequently, his sex drive.

The combined therapies seemed to calm Jan and to direct his attention away from his obsession with young girls. It was impossible, though, to judge the long-term effects of the treatment, or to predict what might happen when the drug therapy was stopped. Dr Jonas was reasonably confident that something approaching a cure would result. Others were not so hopeful.

'Paedophiles always slip back into their old ways,' said a colleague of Jonas's from Indianapolis. 'They're exactly like heroin addicts, they can't leave it alone. The fundamental problem with every single one of them is a flawed personality and low capacity for self-discipline. No amount of behavioural treatment or drug-suppression is going to make any long-term improvement. Even castration doesn't change them. The only answer, in the end, is to keep them shut away so they don't harm children. The alternative to *that*, which I don't necessarily condone, is to keep them sedated at all times, or execute them.'

13
Antisocial Personality

The Antisocial Personality Disorder has been described as a pattern of continuous and chronic antisocial behaviour which consistently violates the rights of other people. It includes conscious and unconscious conflicts and various defence mechanisms. There is usually a marked absence of sympathetic feelings and remorse.

'In my experience more rubbish is talked about this so-called condition than any other,' said a London barrister. 'Another name for the Antisocial Personality Disorder is bullying. This is an example of psychiatry wandering off its turf and getting involved with things that don't concern it.'

Many psychiatrists say that it is easy to distinguish between plain thuggery and the pathological league of anti-social acts, and they point out that the four main criteria for a diagnosis of Antisocial Personality Disorder are particularly clear in sufferers where they are prominent to an extent well beyond the character-trait boundaries of rebels and malcontents. The key clinical features are:

1. Inability to make loving relationships
2. Unpremeditated behaviour
3. Absence of guilt with marked callousness
4. Failure to be improved by experience.

'I couldn't have given a better description of the classic bully,' commented the barrister when he was shown the list. 'Over and over we see this, the listing and cataloguing of degenerate character traits, lumped together under a contrived heading, inflated with jargon and served up as clinical conditions.'

The barrister denied that he was simply unsympathetic to psychiatry and its practitioners. His objections, he insisted, were aimed mainly at 'clinical claim-jumpers, who habitually appropriate certain areas of plain criminal behaviour and turn it into mental illness.'

The case which follows is held, by some, to demonstrate the Antisocial Personality Disorder with particular clarity. Others have viewed it as no more than the repellent history of a hopeless degenerate.

CASE STUDY: *Thoroughly Rotten . . .*
Eleven days after his twenty-second birthday Jackson Lowe was taken before a court near his home town of Manning, Texas, to answer charges on three counts of burglary. The prosecution would show that a man answering Lowe's description, who left behind partial fingerprints closely matching Lowe's, had broken into two homes and a factory on consecutive nights and stolen goods and cash to a value of eleven hundred dollars.

Lowe was a handsome young man, fashionably hard-eyed and surly looking, with a shock of sun-bleached ginger hair that hung in a quiff over one eye. To the dispassionate observer he looked like a none-too-smart young Texan of a type replicated, with only minor variations, across the entire state.

'From his looks,' a police officer said later, 'Lowe was just an ordinary young guy that got burnt having a dabble at crime. A wild boy, I suppose, but again, from the look of him, he was one that would settle down soon enough.'

But at the hearing, which lasted two days, a psychiatrist called by the defence said that Lowe was suffering from a very serious antisocial personality disorder. 'The signs are so clearly defined as to be unmistakable,' the psychiatrist told the court. 'The prisoner is from a family background of acute disharmony and violence. He has a record of serious conduct-disorder from roughly age ten. He was a persistent truant, he ran away from home, he stole even when there was no apparent need to, he was destructive to property, was involved in a number of instances of fire-setting, and behaved cruelly towards smaller children and animals . . .'

The list of juvenile misdemeanours went on and on without any apparent break, said the psychiatrist. It was evident to an experienced observer that Jackson Lowe had sidled into society with certain disadvantages that discoloured his outlook. They left him wide open to negative influences and directed him along a crooked path. His antisocial behaviour had escalated, unchecked, until most of his tendencies were either wayward or downright criminal.

'Nowadays, the accused consistently fails to conform to normal social and lawful behaviour. He is a chronic malefactor. It's as if he had no instinct for fitting in with society. By nature he is aggressive, irritable and short-tempered. He keeps getting in fights, conflict is like a magnet for him. He can hardly ever plan anything ahead of time, and on the few occasions when he does, he invariably falls down on the arrangements. I can cite many other clear signs from Jackson Lowe's recorded behaviour that classify him as suffering from an antisocial personality disorder.'

Lowe was, the psychiatrist concluded, a young man in serious need of intensive, long-term professional treatment.

An earlier evaluation, made by a clinical psychologist when Lowe was twenty, had concluded that he was a malevolent, incorrigible, backsliding criminal quite beyond the reach of any useful treatment, apart from prolonged imprisonment for the protection of the public. This assessment was not made available at the time of the trial for burglary. Nevertheless, the prosecuting attorney appeared to have formed much the same opinion as the psychologist, and he presented the court with a picture of Jackson Lowe as a hard-faced thug without a useful or halfway worthy feature to redeem him.

'Far from being the wounded lamb the defence psychiatrist would have you believe,' he told the court, 'Jackson Lowe is a monster in the making, and I am confident this will not be his last appearance before a court on criminal charges.'

The jury at Manning found Lowe guilty of the three burglaries. The judge awarded him a three-year stretch in the state prison at Huntsville. He served two years and three months and was released in January 1984.

In Huntsville Lowe had fallen in with a long-term prisoner, Bud Mills, who also came from Manning and had lived there in a trailer with his young wife until 1983, when he was arrested on charges of armed robbery and sentenced to twenty years in prison. Lowe promised that when he got out he would look up Mills's wife, Dorothy. He would check that she had no serious problems and reassure her that Bud was in good spirits and hoping for an early parole.

In the event Lowe made immediate sexual advances to Dorothy Mills. She did not resist. Ten days after their first meeting Lowe moved into the trailer with her.

'A lot of people wouldn't understand how it was with us,' Dorothy later explained in a police statement. 'It wasn't love or anything like that. There was none of the clammy possessive stuff, it was a no-commitment thing – he liked sex and somebody to hold on to when he went to sleep. Me too. I'll tell you straight, marriage was more than I ever needed. What I had with Jackson Lowe was just right.'

On the evening of 12 January they were on the couch in front of the TV, eating pizza and drinking beer. Lowe had been quiet for several minutes when suddenly he slapped the arm of the couch and leaned forward. He looked at Dorothy. There was an uncharacteristically earnest glint in his eyes as he told her he had come to a decision. Instead of running crazy risks that kept getting him in trouble, from now on he would earn his living the safest, simplest way anybody could imagine.

'And how's that?' Dorothy asked him.

'Robbing old ladies,' he told her.

Later, in a taped interview with a psychiatrist, Dorothy explained the logic behind Lowe's career move. 'He said it'd be easy and clean and no stress at all. He'd just take their money, nothing else. Goods always got him in trouble before, goods could be traced, and sometimes the people he sold them to would talk to the police. Money didn't need any middle men and old ladies always had money, he reckoned, and I guess he was right. They squirrel it away, they don't trust banks.'

Within twenty-four hours of getting his new idea, Lowe was in the rear garden of a bungalow in a quiet residential district on the other side of town. He had followed an old woman back there from a nearby shopping mall. For an hour he stayed in the bushes in her garden, watching her go about her domestic rituals, noticing that apart from a cat and a parakeet, she lived alone.

It was growing dark when the woman sat down to a meal in the kitchen, talking to the cat all the time she ate, sharing her food with it. When she had washed the supper dishes and put them away, she sat on the couch in her living room, watching television. After five minutes she appeared to fall asleep. Lowe later described what he felt when he realised he could let himself into the house and rob the old woman without any fear of resistance or repercussion.

'It was like a power trip. Even if she hadn't been sleeping, if she'd woken up, she would be helpless, right? She was little and old, I could have broken her with one hand if I needed to do that. But her sleeping like that, there was no threat, the job was such a complete pushover. I stayed out there shivering in the garden a lot longer than I had to, tripping on the feeling, knowing I'd be able to do just anything I wanted with nobody coming back at me.'

The back door was unlocked. Lowe let himself in and went straight to the kitchen where he had seen the old woman leave her purse. He helped himself to $65. He found another $23 in a vase in the hall and a jar full of nickels and dimes in the bedroom. Checking that the old woman was still asleep, he left the house the way he had come in.

Next evening he followed another old woman home and narrowly avoided being savaged by her dog when he crept into the house through a side window. Shaken but determined the evening would not be a loss, he broke into another house, found it empty and took off with nearly $80 from a kitchen drawer.

'The new gimmick of taking only money, and only from

safe targets, really pleased him,' Dorothy Mills said. 'He didn't get all tense and uptight before a job, not like Bud always used to do. It was just like he was going out for a drink. And a bonus for me was he always came back horny.'

Several times in taped interviews Jackson Lowe admitted to being sexually aroused at the scenes of his thefts. He believed it had something to do with the sense of power.

'It was there every time, it wasn't something I could just ignore. I would get a hard-on and it would stay until I did something about it.'

The pattern began to change when he had been stealing from the homes of old women for nearly a month. He still took only money, but he began damaging the premises before he left.

'I don't know why I started doing that. It was just an urge, you know? And it always came at me, even if I'd decided ahead of time I wouldn't let it. I'd get the dough, and when I knew the job was over I would do something, break something or tear up the curtains, or maybe worse than that. One time I poured kerosene all over the kitchen floor. I tried to light it but it wouldn't catch. A car pulled into next door's driveway while I was trying so I got out of there.'

It became clear to Lowe that having adopted a direction and procedure in crime where there were practically no risks, he was now quite deliberately introducing them. A number of times he was nearly identified because he stayed behind after completing a theft to commit some act of vandalism.

One rainy evening he slid in through the back door of a dark old cottage and stood in the passageway, dripping water, watching the old lady who lived there as she made her preparations to go to bed. As she closed the bedroom door and switched out the light, Jackson crept forward to enter the living room and slipped on the puddle that had gathered at his feet. He fell back and cracked his head on the wall. He was dazed, his consciousness fading for a minute, but he was aware that he was on the floor and trying to raise himself.

When his head and his eyes cleared he found himself staring up at the old woman. The hallway light was on and she was pointing a revolver at his forehead. Jackson pushed himself to his feet, sliding up along the wall, making a pleading face, seeing the old woman get close to panic as he moved, her finger tight on the trigger.

'Please don't shoot me,' he recalled saying to her, standing half bent against the wall. 'I came in by mistake, out of the rain. I thought it was somewhere I could shelter, I didn't know anyone lived here.'

The tension seemed to leave the old woman instantly. She believed him. More than that, she began at once to look contrite and apologetic. She put down the gun on the hall table and put out a hand to help Lowe stand upright. In that instant he was filled with a towering anger. He rose to his full height and punched her square in the face with his bunched fist. As she fell he hit her again, hearing a bone in her face break. She lay still, her face turned to the floor.

In the living room Lowe ransacked a bureau and found approximately $20. He put the money in his pocket, then ripped down the curtains and tipped out the tropical fish tank on to the floor. On the way out, he paused in the hallway and kicked the unconscious woman several times on the back and chest.

Two days later a small piece appeared in a local paper reporting that an old lady had been savagely attacked in her home. She had subsequently undergone fourteen hours of surgery to repair a punctured lung. It had not been possible for the surgeons to save the sight of her left eye, which had been destroyed by a splinter of cheekbone penetrating the eyeball from beneath.

Shortly afterwards, on the night of 20 March, Lowe crept on to the wide veranda outside the home of Inge Smart, a retired school teacher rumoured to keep a large amount of cash at home. Lowe watched for a while as the seventy-one-year-old widow slept in an armchair in her living room. When he was sure she was properly asleep, he cut through the screen door with a pocket knife and let himself in. He went quietly to the bedroom where, in the bottom of a closet and in a couple of bureau drawers, he found and pocketed $760 in small-denomination bills sealed in a number of old charity-appeal envelopes.

When he got back to the living room Inge Smart was still asleep. Lowe knew perfectly well that he could have walked out of the house right then and he would never have been connected with the theft.

But in line with what had become standard procedure, he did not leave. He stood over the sleeping woman, staring at her placid face for several minutes, aware things were changing again. He listened to the regular hiss of her breathing, watching the trace of the carotid pulse in her neck. Then he began punching her on the head and face. He kept at it for almost a minute, he believed, pulping her nose, fracturing her jaw and inflicting catastrophic damage on her brain.

In the bathroom he washed the blood off his hands and arms, then went back to the living room. Inge's body lay spread-eagled on the floor, blood leaking from her nose and ears. As Lowe stared at her again he saw her hands twitch. He got down on his hands and knees, listened at her broken mouth and realised she was still breathing. He took a cushion from the armchair and pressed it hard over her face, suffocating her. Then, when he was sure she was dead, he had sexual intercourse with her body.

Two hours later, bathed and wearing clean clothes, Jackson Lowe drove off with a friend for a night on the town. Inge's body was tied up in a blanket in the back of the car. At a liquor store on their way, where an assistant recalled seeing Lowe ostentatiously showing off a roll of bills, they bought a bottle of Jack Daniel's and headed on to the nearest large town.

'The pair of them were hooting and giggling,' the store assistant recalled, 'like two guys that had smoked more Mary-Jane than was conducive to moderate behaviour.'

Five miles down the road from the liquor store they threw Inge's body into a dense patch of shrubbery near the roadside. It was found next morning, and a week later Jackson Lowe was arrested for the robbery and murder.

At his trial the defence called Dr Lawrence Skelton, the psychiatrist who had warned a jury, almost three years earlier, that Lowe was in urgent need of treatment. This time Skelton was even more forceful in asserting that this prisoner had a desperately serious mental illness which was growing steadily worse.

'He is caught in this affliction of his and is under its control. He does not have the freedom of choice which is natural to most sane beings.'

Skelton had dug extensively into Jackson Lowe's background, studying old medical and probation records, interviewing teachers, employers, relatives and male and female friends, including Dorothy Mills. The picture that emerged,

Skelton insisted, was unmistakably that of a man with severely disordered instincts and uncontrolled impulses. He was literally powerless to deflect himself from a downward spiral of antisocial behaviour that would destroy him if it continued unchecked.

'It began early,' Skelton told the court. 'His parenting experience was loveless and was characterised mainly by neglect.'

Lowe was an only child. His mother, an unmarried teenager at the time he was born, had made it clear she did not want the child. She ran away and left him when he was three. A succession of aunts, a grandmother and one sexually-abusing male cousin provided young Jackson with a haphazard, offhand upbringing entirely devoid of affection or guidance. He was permitted near-total freedom and was only rebuked or punished if his behaviour caused trouble for other members of the family.

'He suffered profound emotional deprivation,' Dr Skelton went on, 'and that led inevitably to a lowering of his self-esteem, and to consequent unconscious anger. Lacking moral example and guidance, he had no notion of the usual barriers, his perceptions of right and wrong were deficient. His conscience was so seriously underdeveloped it hardly existed at all. He was and is able, in his subterranean anger, to commit antisocial acts without a measurable trace of guilt.'

A childhood pattern of petty crime had hardened into criminality by the time Lowe was sixteen, Skelton said. He burgled shops and homes, forged cheques and regularly adopted aliases to obtain goods on credit. Increasingly he used his rugged good looks to ingratiate himself with women and then steal from them. On four occasions he had become violent when challenged by suspicious traders, and he actually broke the leg of one man who tried to stop him leaving a store.

'All of that,' said Skelton, 'was the background to the career of thefts from elderly women, culminating in the night when Jackson Lowe stepped on to the veranda outside Inge Smart's home.'

Questioning the psychiatrist, the prosecution attorney asked if it was not a sign of plain depravity that Lowe compounded a simple robbery with brutal murder and sexual assault of the corpse.

'And having done that,' the attorney went on, 'he tried for a time to convince the police that it was his friend who beat the old woman so savagely, that it was the same friend who had sex with her dead body. Would you not agree that is the behaviour not of a mentally sick man, but of a moral bankrupt?'

'I accept that Jackson Lowe did those terrible things, and that he tried to shift the blame to someone who regarded him as a friend,' said Dr Skelton. 'Jackson did all that because it is consistent with the pattern within which he is trapped. He is caught in a matrix of profoundly antisocial behaviour, it's what characterises his illness. He cannot escape that pattern on a whim or an impulse of his own – he can only do it with the help of prolonged and intensive psychiatric treatment.'

To counter the defence plea for a sympathetic judgement, the prosecution called on the expert opinion of Dr Reginald Barton, a forensic psychiatrist who has interviewed, at length, more than 1,400 murderers. In Barton's stated view, Jackson Lowe was a 'thoroughgoing sociopath, to whom killing someone is not a matter for guilt or any sense of wrongdoing.'

Dr Barton was just as direct with his prognosis. 'There

is no cure for this kind of individual,' he said, 'because there is not in any real sense an illness. He will never be any better than he is, and if his movements are not forcibly restricted he will go on doing harm.'

The conflicting views of the two psychiatrists were aired through several more minutes of rebuttal. Skelton maintained that Jackson Lowe's condition was obvious to anyone with even the most rudimentary skills in psychiatric evaluation. 'Lowe's charming surface, coupled to his underlying callousness, is itself a classic symptom of the antisocial personality disorder.'

All of Lowe's symptoms and signs, countered Barton, were those of a nasty personality that certain theory-worshippers were just longing to hang a psychiatric interpretation on. Barton further pointed out that millions of children survived worse upbringings than Jackson Lowe's, and came out of the experience unmarked.

In closing statements the defence pleaded for humane understanding of a mind overthrown by evil social circumstances, while the prosecution reminded the jury that real mental illness and fashionable claptrap were quite different from one another and were easily distinguishable. All the members of the jury had to do was apply their common sense.

The jury took only eighty minutes to convict Jackson Lowe of capital murder, for which there are just two possible sentences in Texas: life imprisonment or death. Three so-called Special Issues determine whether or not the convicted party deserves to die. There must be unanimous agreement among the jurors that the murderer deliberately and with full intent killed his victim; second, there has to be a probability, attested to by an expert, that the defendant would commit criminal acts in the future, making him a continuing threat to society; third, no evidence of reasonable cause or provocation can be produced to mitigate the defendant's homicidal behaviour.

It is the second issue, the question of future behaviour, that forms the core of Texas life-or-death courtroom tussles. This issue permits juries to sentence a defendant to death not merely for a crime or crimes he has committed, but in the light of crimes he might arguably commit at a later time.

To help influence the jury in its separate deliberations and decide whether Jackson Lowe should die or be sentenced to life imprisonment, the defence again called Dr Skelton. He made an earnest plea for clemency, telling the court that the man in the defendant's chair was in every real sense an invalid, who could not be any more ill if he had leprosy heaped on what he was already suffering.

'He displays all four of the classic symptoms of a person suffering from a crippling antisocial personality disorder.' Skelton held up his fingers and counted on them. 'One, he perpetually fails in his attempts to make loving relationships. Two, he is chronically impulsive in his actions. Three, he lacks any sense of guilt, and four, he has failed to learn from any of his adverse experiences. These are the stigmata of a serious sickness, and we have a duty to treat the sick, not to destroy them.'

Before leaving the stand Dr Skelton said he agreed that the public should be protected from Jackson Lowe as long as he remained dangerous. But he insisted that the prisoner's life was worth saving, and that Lowe could even yet make a useful contribution to society.

The prosecution brought back Dr Reginald Barton. He was asked whether, in his expert opinion, Lowe was really as sick as Dr Skelton claimed.

'In my view, he isn't sick at all. There's an unfortunate

belief among too many psychiatrists that if a person does wrong, then he must be mentally disturbed in some way. It's my experience that most of the murderers I've dealt with were not suffering from any mental illness whatsoever.'

'So what was wrong with them, Doctor?'

'They were just rotten individuals.'

The defence objected to that evaluation, but Barton countered that it was a lot more valid than claiming that a history of evil-doing could be passed off as a diagnosis of severe mental illness.

'And would you say, from your position of unrivalled expertise,' the prosecution attorney continued, 'that Jackson Lowe is a rotten individual like those others?'

'Thoroughly rotten,' Dr Barton said. 'The man doesn't have a decent motive or sentiment in his entire malignant nature. He has no regard for common decencies, or for the rights of other people.'

And in Dr Barton's expert opinion, was Lowe likely to kill again?

'He most certainly is. To him, killing the old lady was not much different from trying out a new brand of beer. He liked it, so he's likely to have some more.'

Defence counsel argued strenuously that Dr Barton's evidence was no more than highly subjective opinion unsupported by any scientific proof. So the prosecution asked Dr Barton again.

'Doctor, could you give us your opinion, from the standpoint of a trained forensic psychiatrist with many years' experience – will Jackson Lowe, if he is imprisoned and eventually paroled, commit criminal acts of violence against innocent members of the public?'

'Yes sir,' Dr Barton said stiffly, 'I have a solid opinion in the matter you elucidated.'

'What is your opinion, then?'

'That there is not a shadow of doubt that Jackson Lowe, who has been a criminal since boyhood, whose evil behaviour has grown worse as the years have passed and has resisted all efforts at correction, will commit further acts of violence in the future if he is set free to do so.'

The jury took ten minutes to decide unanimously that Jackson Lowe should be put to death by lethal injection.

14
Kleptomania

The central feature of Kleptomania is a persistent failure to resist stealing things when there is no need for them, and no desire to profit from the theft. Very often the stolen items are given away immediately, or discarded in public litter bins. At other times they are hoarded, or buried, or taken back and left in the shops where they were stolen.

Kleptomania is classified as a compulsive disorder, and like other compulsions it is typified by growing tension before the act, gratification immediately afterwards, then a lessening of tension, sometimes with remorse and depression, sometimes without. The thefts are not planned and no accomplices are ever involved. There is rarely any daredevil element to the stealing, but Kleptomaniacs do not always consider the possibility of being caught. One point of diagnosis is especially clear: if a stolen object is the goal of a theft, then it is not a case of Kleptomania, because in Kleptomania the object of the exercise is solely the act of stealing.

Kleptomania is not particularly common, although it is

probably more widespread than the records show. Fewer than five per cent of arrested shoplifters have a history consistent with the disorder. Even among those who fit the diagnosis, it is likely that a number of offenders have falsified their histories to suit the disorder. There are no figures for the sex ratio in Kleptomania, but since shoplifting is more common among women than men, it is likely there are more female Kleptomaniacs than males.

Some investigators have insisted that Kleptomaniacs are motivated by a powerful psychic sexual drive, while others believe the motivation is completely – or at least largely – aggressive. Analysts who put importance on symbolism see substantial meaning in the act of stealing itself. According to one extraordinary theory from an American analyst, the thief bypasses the buying process so that he or she gets hold of a valuable object complete with its 'pure' character, (pure because it is unsold, so it is unsmirched by commerce), and the act of theft therefore symbolises a need to obtain something of untarnished value to replace, symbolically, some 'quality shortfall' in the Kleptomaniac's personality.

Kleptomania is often found in conjunction with other psychological disorders, such as depression, anorexia nervosa, bulimia nervosa, and – especially among females – pyromania. Kleptomania, even in people with no other obvious disorders, tends to surface at times of emotional stress.

CASE ONE: *A Thrilling Tension*

In 1990 a series of thefts of valuable miniature china ornaments from a Berlin department store prompted the management to step up the security coverage of the small sales area from which the ornaments were being taken.

'It was no bigger than ten metres square,' a police officer said, 'a corner of the fancy goods floor, easy to police, and not exactly crowded at any time. The store management set up a wide-angle TV camera linked to a video recorder, and store detectives circulated regularly. The thefts, however, continued. The videotapes showed nothing suspicious and the detectives had no cause to suspect any of the customers who browsed in the area. During one six-day period, two ornaments a day were being taken.'

The management began to see the thefts as a grim challenge. A year before, they had been targeted by animal-rights groups because they sold fur garments; a certain amount of understandable paranoia now fuelled a drive to get this latest attack on their operation cleared up as fast as possible.

They set up a second camera, positioned to view the fancy goods department from the opposite angle to the first, and detectives were put on an overlapping patrol, so that one did not leave the area until another moved in. The thefts continued.

'They began to wonder if somebody had something against the particular brand of ornaments being taken,' the police officer said. 'They decided to put all of that particular manufacturer's items into locked glass cases. But almost immediately, the thefts switched to another make of ornaments.'

Three weeks after the thefts began, the police had a call from the owner of a modest bric-à-brac shop in the south of the city. He was bewildered, he said, because he had lately noticed that valuable and apparently brand new porcelain ornaments were turning up in his shop.

'He was finding them in odd places,' the police officer said, 'like at the backs of crowded shelves, in bargain bund-

les and sitting on the window ledge. They were the ornaments stolen from the department store.'

A police watch was put on the bric-à-brac shop and
within three hours a woman was caught depositing two
little ornaments in a second-hand cigarette box. She did
not appear surprised when she was caught; in fact she
displayed no emotion at all and went away quietly with the
police officers. She was well-to-do, something of a socialite
and lived in one of the most prosperous areas of Berlin.
When she had been charged with the thefts, all of which
she freely admitted, a forensic psychiatrist interviewed her
and found her as cooperative as she had been with the
police.

'She had been happily married, or so she believed, for
thirty-two years,' the psychiatrist said, 'and then, like a
hammer blow from nowhere, her husband left her for a
woman less than half her age. She was devastated, under-
standably, and for a time she withdrew into herself, cancelling all her social engagements, seeing no one. About a
year later, she decided it was time she faced the world
again. She decided to ease herself back into society and
began by turning up for lunch at a fashionable restaurant.
She observed that although acquaintances acknowledged
her, and were pleasant, they were a good deal less *glad* to
see her than she had expected. As she put it, she hadn't
imagined they would be ecstatic, but she believed there
would have been the odd tear, and a hug or two. But her
return was not greeted with any discernible emotion.
People were warm enough, but they were polite.

'Thinking it over afterwards she realised, slowly, that she
was now that most awkward of social creatures, the middle-
aged woman on her own. Her friends, now that she needed

them more than ever, would never be as warm towards her as they had been in the past. That made her profoundly sad.'

The woman had considerable strength of character, however, and she set about restructuring her social life. She made a point of behaving in a much cooler manner with friends, so that her acceptance of a solo existence would be signalled; she dragooned cousins and nephews into taking her to the theatre, to dinner and to sundry events on the social calendar. She made herself adopt the practice of auto-sustenance – 'being a light unto myself'.

One day, while buying gloves in a department store, she had a sudden and powerful urge to steal something. She was surprised at herself, though not shocked, and she had to admit it had been a long time since she had experienced such a thrilling tension. In the end she stole a leather wallet and hurried out of the store with it. She was shaking all over and felt a great sense of accomplishment. That same evening she put the wallet in an envelope and posted it back, anonymously, to the department store.

'After that,' the psychiatrist said, 'she stole something nearly every day, though never without feeling compelled to do it. Her own insight into her behaviour suggested that this was her sex life and social life rolled into one. The stealing compensated for those parts of her existence that were now missing. She felt rather good for a time, and then she realised that because she was so well known, and because she was so obviously prosperous, no one would ever suspect her of stealing, even if she did it under their noses. The exercise, she now believed, was largely academic. There was no risk. There was no challenge, either, and that seemed to be even more important.'

As soon as she began setting herself targets, the thefts took on a new excitement. She would still only steal when the urge overtook her – but whenever it did, she had a plan ready. For a time the scheme was to move expensive crystal goblets, one by one, from the glassware department of a store to the china department. This she managed to do, and even enjoyed the spectacle of a puzzled assistant in the china department beginning to discover glass goblets all over the place. After that she moved to another store and began not only moving glass to the china department, but putting china in the glass department, doubling her chance of being caught at the mischief, but also doubling the amusement value of her daily exercise.

'The trouble now,' the psychiatrist said, 'was that she wasn't really stealing anything, and after a time she felt dissatisfied again. So she went back to the practice of actually removing items from the stores. She had been doing that for a couple of weeks when she got the idea of trying to remove a large exclusive store's entire stock of a particular kind of ornament. It would be quite an undertaking, she knew, so she planned everything with care. With an almost *psychotic* degree of care, I'd say.'

Still the central motivating factor was the woman's compulsive urge to steal. For all her planning and scheming, the act itself was what mattered, her joy (that was the word she used) was in the moment of achieving the illicit goal, the taking of the object. She believed that the plotting and the setting of targets fulfilled some minor deficit in her life since her husband had left her, but it was something unconnected with the urge to steal and probably quite minor.

'The way she got the ornaments out of the store without being spotted was brilliant,' the psychiatrist said. 'I don't know if the people at the store ever noticed that the ornaments stolen were always taken from near the edge of the display tables, but they were – they had to be.'

The woman entered the store each day in disguise. She did more than resort to a simple change of clothes and a wig; she disguised herself thoroughly. When she played an old woman, she tied a length of cord between her knees, so that she could only take short steps, and she would wear a scarf folded several times under her dress at the shoulders, to simulate a stoop. She told the psychiatrist she spent hours on make-up, being completely sure she was unrecognisable before she set foot outside her house.

'Even then, if she was in a store, covered in make-up that took ages to apply, wearing shoes that made her hobble and clothes she would not normally be caught dead in, if she didn't get the urge to steal, the thrilling, part-frightening anticipation, then she went home without even trying. That did not happen often, however.'

The method of stealing the ornaments was the only legacy from her husband for which she was grateful. He was a theatrical director and had often taught the principles of movement and body-emphasis to seminars at which his doting wife had been present. She knew that a large movement of the hand or arm draws attention from a smaller movement of the other hand or arm. The value of body cover for a necessary manoeuvre – the example her husband had always given was a sword stuck in its sheath – was known to her too; she had used it a few times during minor social emergencies when a button came undone, or one occasion when a stocking began to slide down her leg.

'She would reach out momentarily to touch an ornament high on a display, and with the elbow of the opposite arm she would knock another ornament off the table on to the floor. Except it didn't hit the floor, it went into a cushioned velvet bag she let down from under her skirt on a string as she approached the table. The string was at her waistband, and the bag weighted, so it descended softly under its own weight, and lay with its wired-open mouth upwards waiting for an ornament to land in its cushioned interior. Then, as the woman walked away she would take a handkerchief from her waistband, or on some occasions from a pocket, and the action of raising the handkerchief would draw up the string again, since she had grasped the two together. The bag vanished up into the folds of her skirt. On these occasions she always wore long skirts, of course.'

With the coming of the surveillance camera the woman felt an even stronger tension and thrill as she moved in to commit her thefts. She never entered the fancy goods department more than once on any day, and she did not stay longer than two minutes at the most. Fully conscious of the camera's direction and angle of view – again, she was using her husband's techniques, staying aware of the spectator's sight-line – she would position herself so that the arm doing the dirty work was not even visible at the time the move was made.

'The arrival of the second camera stumped her, but only for a short time,' the psychiatrist said. 'She swept past the fancy goods department, held a mental picture of the cameras' points of view, and as she pretended to browse elsewhere she worked out her strategy. She decided she would use another customer for cover and steal the ornament the way she always did.

'It worked. The woman waited until her right side was obscured by another customer between her and the second camera, then she reached out in a broad gesture with her left hand, knocked an ornament off the table with her right elbow, walked off hoisting the bag into her skirts, and was gone – only to return later and do it again in another disguise.'

The idea of leaving the ornaments in the bric-à-brac shop was a whim, a way of disposing of them that did no harm and, the woman felt, added a suitably light touch to the whole business. She said she should have realised there was a chance of being discovered using the little shop.

The case never went to court. Instead, the management of the store came to an arrangement with the woman: she would promise to stop using their shop, and she would make a substantial donation to a charity designated by them. She agreed, and the matter was forgotten.

'The last time I spoke to her was on a follow-up interview,' the psychiatrist said. 'She didn't have to agree to it, but she did. I asked her how she was coping with the compulsion to steal, and she said it was as strong as ever. "I would never have believed it of myself," she said. "But it is only a short time ago that I would never have believed, either, that my husband would leave me. So there we are. Surprises all round. Were it not for the one, there would not be the other." '

The psychiatrist believed that parting remark was the best evaluation of cause and effect in this case that anyone was likely to make. When the woman was leaving the psychiatrist asked her if nowadays she ever had the urge to steal, or gave into random Kleptomaniac impulses. She simply shrugged and smiled.

CASE TWO: *The Power of Guilt*

A doctor in general practice found that on odd occasions he would walk into large Manchester stores like Marks and Spencer's, WH Smith's or Woolworth's, with no other purpose than to steal whatever came to hand. He would not pause or hesitate: the impulse took him, he strode into the store, took whatever he could, and marched smartly back out again. He always threw away the items he took, or, when appropriate, he gave them to children playing near houses where he made his calls.

'He came to the hospital and told me about it, and about how scared he was that he'd get caught,' a psychiatrist said. 'This was a severe compulsion. He would come out of one of those shops with something or other clutched in his pocket, and he would be sweating and shaking and downright terrified he'd get jumped on at any second. Yet he couldn't stop himself doing it when the urge took him. The way he described it, he would go into the shop like he was in the grip of something bigger than he was, and he would know he was going to steal something and he would be scared, but, at that point, he would be more excited than scared. He would snatch whatever he could – a pen, an aerosol of deodorant, any damned thing at all really. As soon as he had it the fear came down on him, there was no sense of accomplishment, no pleasure in making the snatch. His fear never made him put the item back, though, he always hung on to it once he had it. And he had to leave the store with it.'

The GP told the psychiatrist how he cried at night, thinking of what he had done, imagining how his career could be ruined by one senseless, pointless act. Then in daylight it was a different pressure he felt, not direct fear and remorse but the imminence, the threatened arrival of a compulsion that he had to stay with until it was carried through to completion.

'There's no hard and fast treatment for someone with Kleptomania,' said the psychiatrist. 'You have to try to find an underlying cause, make them confront it, and that way take away the pressure that drives them into jeopardy. So there we were, him and me, trying to figure out why he did it, why he regularly put his neck on the line the way he did.'

The GP had recently lost his mother, who had died after a long illness. It was some time before he revealed this to the psychiatrist, and when he did he said he doubted if his behaviour could have anything to do with his mother's death. But then the psychiatrist did some simple checking of dates and pointed out that the first time the GP stole from a shop was ten days after his mother died.

'So he had a good long think,' the psychiatrist said. 'I know now the veils clinging to his pain were hard to lift. He didn't come back to see me for a while and I got worried in case he had been arrested or something similarly awful had happened. I telephoned him one evening, asked how it was going and so on, and he said he would like to talk to me any time I was free.'

They met in a pub that evening and the GP told the psychiatrist that he had finally faced a fundamental truth about himself. In facing it, he said, he had managed to cut himself adrift from his sense of purpose for a time. Now he just felt bewildered, and rather anxious.

'He told me he had realised he never liked his mother. It's a hard thing for a lad to admit to himself or to anybody else, whatever age he is. He said he went home after talking to me the last time, he had a couple of stiff drinks to relax him, and then he sat in a chair and thought about his old mother, and realised that on the day she died he had felt a sweeping sense of relief.'

The GP's mother had dominated him throughout his boyhood, had disapproved of his wife and had – he could now admit – harried his beloved father into an early grave.

'He sat there in the pub,' the psychiatrist said, 'and he told me she was a monster. People started staring when he began to cry, but I encouraged him to let rip, it was doing him more good than I ever would.

'He had worked it all out, he told me. All down the years he had kept himself carefully blinkered to the fact that he disapproved of that old woman. He now realised that he had always responded to any uncharitable thought about his mother by reminding himself how much she had done for him. He knew all that stuff by heart, because she had drummed it into him.'

By stages, the GP said, he had looked at areas of his feelings that he had shied from before, and bit by bit he lost his self-deception about his mother. He told the psychiatrist that he now realised his relief at his mother's death – 'at her removal from my life' – had been close enough to the surface to make him want to punish himself for such a shameful emotion.

'And hence the Kleptomania,' said the psychiatrist. 'His lost sense of purpose, his anxiety, they were tail-end stuff, simple side-effects of the restructuring of a large part of his psyche.'

Two years after speaking to the psychiatrist in the pub that evening, the GP had experienced no further compulsion to steal. His life, he reported, was on an even keel, probably for the first time. His lost sense of purpose had returned, completely refurbished.

CASE THREE: *Magpie*

An inventory at the main warehouse of a DIY wholesaler revealed a discrepancy large enough to merit a full-scale investigation. Staff were questioned by police and eventually one man, a sixty-four-year-old foreman with twenty years' service and less than a year to go until retirement, was singled out. Of all the employees he was the only one with full access to every area, including a high-security bay where the most expensive consumer items were stored.

Under questioning, the man eventually broke down and admitted he had been helping himself to goods for some time. He insisted he had not stolen for profit, but the police did not believe that, considering the fact that items from that particular warehouse were of a quality that people would always buy.

'He kept on insisting he hadn't taken anything with gain in mind,' a police officer said, 'but he wouldn't say what he *did* take the stuff for. We'd heard it all before, anyway, but this man did get rather heated, and eventually somebody asked him just what he had done with the gear. "It's at home," he said. So we went to his house. We got the surprise of our lives.'

In three rooms on the upper floor of his house, the man had stored an eleven-year collection of goods from the warehouse, many of the items now discontinued and at least three of them now collectors' items. Oddly, nothing on that scale had ever been reported missing from the warehouse. There were 270 cans of paint, 16 sets of step ladders, 3 lawnmowers, 20 electric drills, several hundred light bulbs, 10 complete boxed sets of patio furniture, 19 coffee percolators, more than 40 doormats, hundreds of packets of nuts, bolts, screwnails and washers, 50 hammers, dozens of screwdrivers and many, many more items; the contents of the three rooms took several days to itemise.

When the man said, again, that he had not stolen the goods for profit, the police believed him.

'And we were dead keen to know why he did take the stuff, since he'd used none of it,' the police officer said. 'But he just shrugged. He hadn't a clue.'

No charges were brought, and the man was eventually referred for psychiatric treatment. He could not tell the psychiatrist why he stole, or how he felt when he stole, or even if there was any special frequency or pattern to his stealing. The diagnosis was finally entered as Kleptomania. The man did not respond to attempts at therapy. He was retired early from his job, and did not come to the notice of the authorities again.

15
Homicide

Homicide is a general term meaning the killing of a human being by another. It has a number of legal classifications, but the three main categories are

murder, which is the unlawful killing of a human being with a premeditated motive;
manslaughter, the unlawful killing of a human being without premeditated malice;
infanticide, the killing of an infant under the age of twelve months.

This chapter concerns itself with murder, with a passing note on infanticide.

The full legal definition of murder was laid down by Sir Edward Coke in the sixteenth century, and was later modified to accommodate changes made by statutes and a number of court decisions:

Subject to three exceptions, the crime of murder is

committed when a person of sound mind and discretion unlawfully kills any reasonable creature in being and under the Queen's peace with intent to kill or cause grievous bodily harm the death following within a year and a day.

The three exceptions reduce a charge of murder to manslaughter, and they are 1. if the accused was provoked, or 2. if he suffered from diminished responsibility, or 3. if he was acting in pursuance of a suicide pact.

In cases where a woman kills her young child, she can be charged with murder or manslaughter, but in special circumstances the charge can be changed to infanticide. Section 1 of the Infanticide Act (1938) says that

where a woman causes the death of her child under the age of 12 months, but at the time the balance of her mind was disturbed by reason of her having not fully recovered from the effects of childbirth or lactation consequent upon the birth of the child, she shall be guilty not of murder but of infanticide.

Two types of infanticide were noted by P. J. Resnick, writing in the *American Journal of Psychiatry*. When a child was killed within twenty-four hours of being born, usually it meant that the child was unwanted, and often the mother was young and feckless but not mentally ill. When the killing happened more than twenty-four hours after birth, in most cases the mother was depressed, and killed the child to avert the suffering she believed would lie ahead. About a third of these mothers also tried to kill themselves.

In England and Wales all people charged with murder are

assessed psychiatrically by a prison doctor, who will usually ask for a second psychiatric opinion. The defence often obtains independent psychiatric advice. The psychiatric report is based on a full physical and psychiatric examination. The psychiatrist reads all the affidavits from witnesses, the statements made by the accused to the police, and any previous medical records and relevant case work done by social workers. Members of the accused person's family, if there are any, are also interviewed.

Murder can result from a number of conditions described and illustrated under separate headings in this book. There is no single predisposing cause, and probably only a minority of murderers are mentally disturbed. The aim of this chapter is to show murder from the position of the forensic psychiatrist, who is obliged not simply to assess a prisoner's state of mind at the time of the crime and later, but to produce a rounded, detailed, and dispassionate picture of a human being whose future is in the balance. The psychiatrist must also emphasise any special circumstances which only a specialist in mental disorder would be likely to detect.

CASE STUDY: *Out of control*

A twenty-eight-year-old window cleaner called Dennis was accused of the murder of three young women over a period of four days in 1974. While awaiting trial he was visited in a remand facility by Sarah, a forensic psychiatrist appointed by the court to make an evaluation of his mental state.

'Dennis's pre-crime stresses were pretty severe,' Sarah said. 'He was a heavy drinker, and this caused trouble with Mum and Dad, because he owed them money and couldn't keep up the repayments, largely because he was drunk most of the time and couldn't work. His wife was giving him a bad time too, because she had to face the landlord over the arrears of rent, she had to manage on very little money, and on top of all that she was feeling sexually unfulfilled, because Dennis had shown no physical interest in her since the birth of their second child.'

Dennis was also having trouble with loan sharks, to whom he owed several hundred pounds. An emissary from the group had already been in touch and assured him his health would suffer if he did not make up the deficit soon. On the night of his first crime, Dennis had a rancorous argument with his father, a row with his wife and another warning from the loan sharks. With fifteen pounds in his pocket, he went to a bar and started drinking heavily.

'It's worth remembering,' said Sarah, 'that his self-esteem at this time was very low. He didn't believe himself capable of any worthwhile accomplishment – he didn't even believe it was worth anyone's while to try helping him, since he had no value and was likely to go bad on any deal, simply because people like him could never do the right thing, even if they wanted to.'

While he worked at getting himself drunk, a woman approached from the other end of the bar. She was young, nineteen, and had been a prostitute for only a few months. She asked Dennis if he needed company and he shrugged. It was not a rejection, she decided, and sat on the stool next to his. Dennis did not offer to buy her a drink so she asked him if he would buy her a snowball. He shrugged again and nodded to the barman, who attended to the order.

'I started asking him about himself, rubbing my knee on his leg, all that kind of thing,' the girl said. 'He began to show a bit of interest after a minute or two. He wasn't drunk but he was heading that way, his eyes were kind of glassy. When he'd bought me another drink he leaned close and asked me if I liked doing it out in the open. I told him I didn't do it any other place. He thought that was funny, and he asked me if I fancied a bit. It kind of dawned on me then that he thought I was just being pally, you know, like I was the local nymphomaniac, he didn't know I was on the game. So I said yeah, I fancied a bit, but it'd cost. He blinked at me and asked me to say that again, so I did. He sat back then and stared at me. His face turned real nasty. He told me he didn't pay no fuckin' tart for a screw, so I told him tough, it was the only way somebody with a face like his would ever get one. Then I pushed off.'

To the prostitute the exchange was a small ripple, one of many false-start transactions. But to Dennis the encounter had been devastating.

'It was bad enough he felt like dirt.' Sarah said. 'But to be thwarted in the middle of a sexual manoeuvre, and then told he was too ugly ever to get sex without paying for it, was like having a hot knife stuck through his shrivelled ego.'

Dennis told Sarah that he was so consumed with anger and a sense of shame that he felt crippled; he said he literally could not get off the bar stool. Finally, when his legs obeyed him again, he left the pub and went along to the street to a wine bar. In there, when they told him they didn't sell draught beer, he bought a bottle of wine and asked a woman drinking alone if she would share it with him.

'Something made me do that, something I didn't usually have, the drive, I suppose,' Dennis said. 'It must have been the girl in the other bar, the mouthy one, that made me try a bit harder. This woman was friendly, she smiled at me and made space at the bar for us. But I didn't like her. I'd talked to her because that other one had as good as said it wouldn't work. But it did work.'

When the wine was finished the woman bought another bottle. They drank that and Dennis asked her bluntly if she fancied having sex with him. She shrugged, then said OK.

'He had cancelled the impact of what the prostitute said to him,' Sarah said. 'But what he hadn't done was reverse the will of that girl. She had withheld herself from him, he couldn't have her, that was the situation. He could have another woman, but that was not the point. The anger that had flared from the encounter with the prostitute was still there, and now it was more focused, it was being fired by a single heat source – his failure to have sex with the other woman, *the one who had mocked him*. Dennis was in a very dangerous frame of mind. His whole pool of emotional energy was taken up with his own hurt feelings and sense of loss, he had no reservoir of emotion where he could entertain feelings of sympathy or compassion for anybody else.'

He left the wine bar with the woman and they crossed a stretch of ground between half-demolished old buildings, heading for a flat open space where she said her car was parked. Halfway there Dennis was overtaken by a surge of impatient lust. He pushed the woman against a wall and began pulling up her clothes. She complained, and as he continued to handle her roughly she hit him on the face and scratched his cheek.

'That duplicated the rejection he already felt,' Sarah said. 'His anger flared out of control and completely took him over.'

He stumbled back from the woman's flailing hands and fell over a pile of rubble. When he stood up he was holding a half brick. He hit the woman with it, on the hands and arms and face, and then on top of her head, over and over, until the howling stopped and her skull became soft under the repeated impact of the brick.

When he stopped he stood bent over in the half light, panting with the exertion, looking at the body lying on the ground. One knee was bent, the other extended, making it seem that she was lying there in a casual pose, unperturbed by what Dennis had done to her. He snatched up an empty beer bottle, forced the dead woman's knees apart and pushed the neck of the bottle into her vagina. He then kicked the bottle the rest of the way into her.

He did not remember getting home and woke up around ten the following morning. He immediately remembered killing the woman, but although he knew it had happened, he felt strangely detached from the event, as if he had merely dreamt it, or read about it happening somewhere else. His wife was sullen, and when he asked her what was wrong now, she told him that if he wanted to treat a woman like an animal, he had better find somebody else to do it with. Somebody who didn't mind that kind of behaviour. It was some time before he was able to coax an explanation from her. Eventually she told him that he had come home staggering drunk, got into bed and forcibly buggered her.

'The news had a huge impact on Dennis,' Sarah said. 'He had never done anything like that before, he had never *wanted* to do it.' Part of him felt like apologising to his wife, but his self-esteem had dipped again, and the abasement of an apology would have been more than he could withstand. He went out, saying he was going to try for a part-time job. At the local pub he picked up the midday edition of the evening paper and looked for a report of the killing, but there was none.

A short time later, when he was sure no one was about,

Dennis went in among the derelict buildings where he had been the night before and incredibly the body was still there. He picked up the handbag, took a small bundle of banknotes from the purse, pocketed them together with some keys, then dropped the bag on the body and immediately began throwing brick and rubble on it. He worked furiously, transferring a small hill of rubbish from one spot to another, an armful at a time, tearing his fingers and skinning his knuckles with the speed and the effort of dislodging the pieces.

When he was finished the body was buried beneath more than a ton of brick, broken paving stones, plaster and other debris. He moved away from the site as carefully as he had gone in, leaving on the far side. Across the way, on a flat stretch of ground, one car stood. He went and looked inside, then took the keys from his pocket and tried one in the door lock. It turned easily. He got into the car and drove five miles to a river bank, where he pushed the car into the water and watched it slowly sink.

'Far from thinking his life was entering a nightmare phase, as some people might,' Sarah said, 'he was boosted by a sense of accomplishment, the first in a long time. He had covered up the crime, he had done it in an efficient and resourceful way, and he had come back from his positive labours with a few pounds in his pocket – twenty-three pounds, to be exact. Dennis felt good, but of course it didn't last.'

That same afternoon, only a few yards from his front door, he was stopped by a man in a leather jacket who said he now had three days in which to put right the arrears on his loan. Presumably to give Dennis a sense of urgency, the man stood heavily on his foot, almost breaking a toe, as he repeated the warning. Dennis limped away to the pub to spend some of the money he had taken from the dead woman's bag.

'He was very worried,' Sarah said. 'There was no chance of getting the instalment, which was something like sixty pounds, by any honest means. Nobody would employ him or advance him money because he was a bad risk, a notorious one. All he could think of was the possibility of stealing enough to cover himself until he got a regular job again. He drank while he thought about that, mulling over the likeliest prospects, and the drinking gradually made his position seem much less desperate than before.'

He went home half drunk, slept in a chair by the fire, then went out again when it got dark.

'I wasn't thinking about money by then,' he told Sarah. 'I was looking for her, the prostitute. I wanted to turn it round, you know? I wanted it to be friendly between us, and I wanted her to say she hadn't meant what she said about me. It mattered to me a lot.'

He did not see the prostitute in the bar where she had been the previous night, but while he was there another woman spoke to him. She was tall and rather aggressive. She asked him where Toni was. He said he didn't know any Toni. She insisted he did, he had been with her in the wine bar last night, the woman had seen them and she had kept out of the way, even though she was Toni's friend, because she didn't want to interfere. And now Toni wasn't at home, hadn't been home since last night in fact, and nobody had seen her.

'The last I saw of her,' the woman added, 'was going out the door with you.'

Dennis supposed, in retrospect, that it had been far too optimistic of him to believe he had drunk two bottles of wine with a woman in a public place without being noticed.

But this accusing presence behind him in the pub seemed, at the time, to be a very unreasonable intrusion.

'The woman was aggressive, she clearly didn't like him, and his reactive dislike of her grew side by side with his fear of her,' Sarah said. 'He could imagine her going straight to the police as soon as she left the pub. He offered to buy her a drink, but she said she didn't want one. She wanted to know where her friend Toni was, Toni who had never stayed away from home all night before. Finally Dennis said he didn't know what she was talking about, he had been with some girl called Mary all night, and not in the wine bar, either. Of course this made the woman even more aggressive.'

Dennis finally stood up and strode out of the pub. He went round to the car park at the back and the woman followed him, as he guessed she would. He knew she was just drunk enough to make a lot of noise so he pretended to give in to her insistence.

'Give me a lift,' he said, 'I'll take you to her. She didn't want anybody knowing she's at my place, that's all.'

The woman looked cagey, Dennis thought, but she showed him to her car, a Mini. As she opened the door and leaned in, clearing the passenger seat of bags and clothing, he went up behind her and punched her hard three or four times on the back of the head. She made a small sound and fell forward into the car. In a panic Dennis cast about for some more effective way of attacking her and saw a broken, rusted Krooklock lying by the wall. He snatched it up and hammered the woman with it, beating her spine and shoulders, then pulled her out of the car so he could hit her on the head. He swung the Krooklock hard, twice, against the side of her skull and the second time he heard the bone crack.

'He entertained a certain feeling, underneath all his self-doubt and lack of pride, that in moments of positive action he was invincible,' Sarah said. 'It had happened when he covered up the body among the rubble, and it happened again as he bundled the woman back into her car. There was no one else in the car park, it was deserted. He shoved the woman across into the passenger seat, pushed her down so her head, which was bleeding freely, was between her knees. Then he got in and drove off.'

Dennis took the car to an old quarry half full of water. He dragged the woman out, laid her on the ground with her legs spread apart, and pushed the broken end of the Krooklock into her vagina. At that point he believed she was still alive, but she made no sound as he forced the implement into her with both hands.

He then found a large boulder, almost too heavy to pick up, and he brought it to where the woman lay. Standing over her, straddling her body, he dropped the boulder on her face. He noticed the body jerked and shuddered for a few moments.

When he was sure she was dead he pushed the boulder off her broken head and rolled the body over the edge of the quarry into the water. She floated, but that did not trouble him; 'It didn't seem to matter,' he told Sarah. He put the car into neutral, released the brake and pushed it down into the quarry. He then walked home, once more feeling energised by the positive, self-protecting action that he had taken.

'The clearly pathological feature of his behaviour,' Sarah said, 'was that he had no remorse or misgivings about having killed the women, either at the time he committed the murders, or later. If anything, he was beginning to see murder as a straightforward and effective expedient. It was a means of attaining an end, with no moral restraints to trouble him.'

It also seemed to Sarah that murder had destroyed mental barriers Dennis hadn't known were there. His untypical sexual behaviour with his wife was repeated that same night, and this time he remembered doing it, indeed actively wanting to do it. During the night, driven forward by something within himself that he told Sarah felt like a motor in his guts which buzzed along his arms and legs, he went along the silent street to the pub where he usually drank. He took with him an axe handle.

After walking around the building a couple of times in the dark, he used the axe handle to break a lavatory window, then climbed in through the gap. When he reached the bar he heard panting and realised the landlord's Alsatian dog was coming at him. As it reached him and leapt up, he hit it on the snout with the axe handle. The animal dropped back, whining, and Dennis followed it, hitting it repeatedly with the heavy implement until it lay dead, its skull smashed.

Sarah noted that this was another moment of ego-boost. 'Killing had worked for him again. He felt good. He began searching for money, finding none but not feeling disheartened. He was up, he was on a high, and the important thing was, he was not being hampered, he had taken positive steps to make sure that was the case. Then, while he was bumping about behind the bar, the landlord's wife walked in and switched on the light.'

Dennis did not hesitate. He came around the bar, seeing her puzzled look as she stood there in her night-dress, staring at the dead dog, its head in a puddle of blood. She looked at Dennis as he approached her. She shook her head, perhaps puzzled by something too far beyond the ordinary to comprehend just yet.

Seeing the woman's naked body silhouetted through the night-dress by the light from the stairway, Dennis knew in advance what he was going to do, though he had no idea why. He hit her with the axe handle on one side of the head and then on the other. She fell to the floor without uttering a sound and lay staring at him. He believed she was stunned. He leaned forward, bent her knees and pushed them apart. Then he pushed the axe handle into her.

'She screamed with the pain,' Sarah said, 'and that startled Dennis. He snatched a heavy glass soda siphon off the bar and began beating her on the face with it. Her facial bones began fracturing after the third or fourth blow, but he kept on until her forehead caved in. He said it felt like he was doing a job, there was no sense of another person being involved.'

When he finished he straightened up and saw the landlord standing in the doorway. The man looked terrified. Dennis stepped back from the dead woman and pointed at the telephone on the wall.

'Maybe you should phone the police,' he said.

In court, Sarah testified to Dennis's detachment when he killed the three women, and his complete lack of remorse or concern over their deaths. She said that various pathological traits could be deduced from the fact that in each case he inserted objects into the women's bodies. There were in fact so many theories about this, however, and the practice was so widespread among murderers, that she felt nothing would be gained by parading the arguments in court.

Concluding her findings, she said that in assessing Dennis's level of dangerousness, she had taken due account of the impulsive nature of his crimes, his difficulty in coping

with stress, his sadistic traits and his general unwillingness
to delay any forms of gratification. In her professional view,
he was a highly dangerous individual and an undoubted
hazard to society at large.

Dennis was found guilty of the three murders and was
given three sentences of life imprisonment. He died in
prison in 1989 of complications arising from an aortic
aneurysm.

16
Pathological gambling

For the majority of people who gamble it is a leisure pursuit offering diversion and an innocent thrill; winnings, when they come, are a bonus. The average person feels no unusually strong attraction to this area of risk-taking. In contrast, there are men and women who spend most of their time and their money on gambling. When they win they bet more heavily, and when they lose all their available cash they will often take other people's, to feed an urge that can develop and grow into a dependence with a hold as powerful as any narcotic.

The inclination to take risks varies from person to person, and many people need risk as a regular feature of their lives. A percentage of them will take up gambling, and a percentage of these, in turn, will gamble pathologically. There have been very few surveys of the subject, but one carried out in 1974 suggested that among people betting on horses and dogs in the UK, more than 80,000 had serious gambling problems. In 1977, a survey of British prisons conducted by the Royal College of Psychiatrists suggested that roughly ten per cent of prisoners had gambling problems. Published estimates for the United States put the figure for pathological gamblers at between two and three per cent of the adult population.

The disorder is more common in men than in women. The fathers of men and the mothers of women with the problem are more likely to suffer from the disorder than the general population. Women who gamble pathologically are more likely than other women to be married to alcoholics who spend a lot of time absent from home. Alcohol dependence among the parents of pathological gamblers is a commoner picture than it is in the population at large.

Pathological gamblers often give the impression of being over-confident, quick-tempered, full of energy and free with their money. They tend to be of the opinion that while money has caused their sometimes disastrous predicaments, more money would solve everything.

Typical complications include the sufferer becoming an outcast from his family, losing his professional and social status, and eventually degenerating into a solitary, often vagrant existence, intermittently joining up with antisocial fringe groups.

The following clinical study describes a typical case.

CASE STUDY: *No future, No past*
Jonathan, a thirty-seven-year-old family doctor attached to a practice in south London, was interviewed by a forensic psychiatrist shortly after he was arrested. He was being held on eight charges ranging from theft to illegal trading in restricted drugs. The psychiatrist, Dr Hibbert, said that when he first saw Jonathan, it was hard to believe he was interviewing a professional man.

'He looked like a tramp. Smelt like one, too. He hadn't shaved for a week or more, his hair was stiff with dirt, his skin had that look the crusties get, a kind of grey sheen from regular neglect, and his clothes stank of urine. When I first tried to talk to him he cried a lot and more or less babbled. He didn't make any sense. He had been drinking tonic wine and it had made him terribly maudlin.'

Jonathan was in better shape the next time he met Dr Hibbert. He was sober, he had been given a shave and a haircut, he was eating solid food without being sick, and the only odour around him was soap and mouthwash. He said he was ready to cooperate as much as he could, and agreed to the interviews being tape-recorded. Talking about his gambling problem he admitted, straight away, that he had been skating on thin ice for three years before he finally lost control of his life.

'The gambling had a hold of me as far back as my second or third year in practice. My wife had left me – it was incredible, we were two years into our marriage, that's all, and she went off with an older colleague. I suppose I took it badly, very badly in fact, although I didn't let it show. I was ambitious, I didn't want any setbacks at that early stage of my career. But my student-days habit of regular gambling came back. Would that be called compensation?'

Dr Hibbert was anxious not to make any judgements on Jonathan's behalf, or to endorse any that were only half formed. Instead, he encouraged Jonathan to analyse his situation to a point where clear answers or at least strong possibilities would emerge. At the same time, Dr Hibbert always believed it was a good idea to nudge the patient in the direction of possible answers, if only to eliminate them.

'Did you have a stable family background, Jonathan? You have an excellent educational record, but that doesn't tell us anything about the kind of home you came from.'

His childhood had been nothing like average, Jonathan said, although he wasn't sure if it had been good or bad. His father, a consultant surgeon, had spent very little time with his three children and when he did put in an appearance, it was usually to discipline one or other of them. The mother drank heavily and died of complications arising from cirrhosis when she was thirty-nine. At that time Jonathan, the oldest child, was thirteen. He was sent to live with his father's sister; his two brothers went to their maternal grandparents, and Jonathan saw very little of them after that.

The aunt he lived with was an eccentric character, a professional compiler of crosswords who was also an inveterate gambler. She was successful insofar as she won more bets than she lost, and she prided herself on her knowledge and understanding of flat racing. A day rarely passed when she did not put on at least one bet, and she had telephone accounts with three bookmakers. She got Jonathan interested in studying form and by the time he was seventeen he was able to place a respectable percentage of winning bets.

'When I was a student, I could double my allowance for the month with a couple of on-the-nose winners,' he said. 'Those were the good days, of course. It was scientific back then, I was detached. When I took to it in earnest, after my wife cleared off, it was more like a disease. Over a period of time I became obsessed. I even began to think about races and racing form while I was dealing with patients. That took time to happen, as I say, but it had an awful inevitability about it. What I mean is, I knew in advance that I was going to get drawn into sick gambling, the compulsive superstitious kind, the nerve-end gambling that gets a hold on you like an itch in your brain. I'd seen it plenty of times in other people, I'd referred two patients suffering from it to psychiatrists. And every now and again I'd been aware that it could happen to me, I knew I could get *too* wrapped up in my gambling.'

Along with the obsessive gambling came a decline in Jonathan's betting skill and an increasing belief in instinct and lucky omens. He would back horses which, on form, were clear losers, believing they had some magical significance in their names, or in variable combinations of their jockeys, their race venues and the times of the month – even the times of the day. The curious thing, he noted, was that this kind of haphazard, superstitious amateurism consumed much more of his time and energy than scientific form-book gambling ever did.

'And of course I began losing. At first it was manageable amounts, thirty or forty pounds a week. But that changed. The more time I spent at it, the bigger the bets became. It reached the point, after a while, that if I had one winner a week, it was an event, and the winnings wouldn't come anywhere near to making up the deficit in my funds. Three years ago, I finally got myself into real trouble.'

His gambling expenses had reached a level where he could not afford to keep up the mortgage on his small house. By a discreet arrangement with the building society he surrendered the property and borrowed privately to cover arrears of approximately £800, over which they had threatened a lawsuit, which would have been socially and professionally damaging. He moved into a small flat over the practice, which suited his partners, since after-hours security at the surgery was a serious concern and there had already been tentative plans to employ a caretaker.

'So I had a roof over my head,' Jonathan said, 'but I

gambled away the last of my money. Thanks to accounts with two bookies, I had gambling debts amounting to three thousand pounds. On top of that, I had borrowed two thousand from my father and a thousand from my brother. To cap it all I began drinking heavily, just like dear old Mum. My situation was frankly terrible, but the facts didn't shock me out of the downward spiral. I went right on gambling with any money I could scrounge on one excuse or another.'

Dr Hibbert noted that Jonathan was describing a disturbance in impulse control which was exactly like dependence on a psychoactive drug. In both cases the addicted person has poor control of his self-destructive behaviour and he carries on with it, disregarding the consequences.

'I discussed the case with a colleague who suggested a diagnosis of Antisocial Personality Disorder,' Dr Hibbert said, 'but that would not have been right, in my view. Jonathan's antisocial behaviour was limited to his drinking and his borrowing money on false pretences. He had no history of antisocial behaviour, and there was no evidence of any blunting of his ability to do his job or to deal with other people. The only signs of impaired functional ability were associated with his betting on the horses. So strictly speaking the diagnosis had to be Pathological Gambling.'

After a time Jonathan's senior partner took him aside and told him, bluntly, that he would have to improve his behaviour, and quickly, if he didn't want to face the alternative of looking for an appointment elsewhere. The other partners had complained about his borrowing, his feeble excuses for not repaying (he owed one partner £300), his practice of turning up for work dishevelled and smelling of drink, and the time he spent away from the practice engaged on mythical house calls and research on a paper he said he was preparing for the *British Medical Journal*.

Jonathan promised to shape up, but carried on exactly as before.

'My mental state at the time was curious,' he told Dr Hibbert. 'I wouldn't dwell on the awfulness of my situation, I simply wouldn't acknowledge it. I wouldn't even admit to myself that there was such a thing as a day-to-day world where such a mess could develop. Everything, my whole life, my awareness, my hope, my focus of understanding, was concentrated into the present.'

He did not have any inclination to think of the future, he said, and it would have been too hellish to contemplate anyway. Similarly he had no reference to the past.

'All I had was the here-and-now. I walled up my awareness, I blinkered my memory and my ability to think ahead even to the next hour. I was a kind of automaton without a trace of apprehension. The need to gamble was the only living, squirming thing inside me.'

When Jonathan could borrow no more money from his partners, he began to steal. At first it was from the practice float, kept in the reception area. Three times he robbed it, meaning to put the money back, but never being able to. Eventually the reception staff refused to have anything further to do with the management of the float, since they had to withstand suspicion and the humiliation of questioning by the senior partner each time it was found short. The money was handled thereafter by the senior partner, so Jonathan no longer had access to the cash box.

'So I began lifting money off patients. Terrible. I cringe thinking about it, but at the time it was a case of needs must when the devil drives. I would make all kinds of excuses to get men to take off their jackets and shirts, trousers too if I could make it plausible, and while they

trotted through to the examination room I would dip into
their wallets or hip pockets. I robbed women too, of course.
With them it was easier, really, for all they had to do was
leave the handbag on my desk, although women tend to
carry a lot less cash than men, I found.'

Jonathan believed it was his acute desperation for money
that guaranteed the success of these thefts. When he was a
boy he had read somewhere that a burning need and an
unwillingness to accept defeat were twin drives that nearly
always guaranteed success. He was now convinced of that.
His own experience made him understand how a junkie
could successfully steal goods and money to a value of
sometimes a hundred pounds, *every day*, in order to feed
his habit.

'At first I was discreet, just a few pounds from each
selected patient, or nothing at all if they weren't carrying
much. I didn't want to arouse suspicion, even though it
would have been pretty far-fetched, I suppose, for someone
to imagine his doctor had picked his pocket.'

After a while discretion was discarded. Bookmakers
began to press Jonathan for their money. Gambling debts
cannot be recovered by law, but alternative methods used
by some bookies are more effective than those available to
the police and bailiffs. Jonathan was stopped in the street
as he was getting into his car and told bluntly that his fingers
would be broken if he did not put a sizeable instalment of
one outstanding debt in the hands of his creditor within
twenty-four hours.

'I needed a hundred and fifty pounds,' Jonathan said. 'I
still didn't think ahead, but I sweated on the bone-instinct
of what lay ahead unless I paid up.'

That afternoon, during a particularly busy session at the
surgery, he stole nearly two hundred pounds. Half of it
came from patients' jackets, trousers and bags, the rest was

from the pocket inside a partner's Filofax, which he had left on his desk while he was out of the office. Next day Jonathan paid the instalment on his debt. He felt a buzz of elation at so closely avoiding disaster; to celebrate, he blew the rest of the money on one silly, impulsive bet on a twelve-to-one outsider.

'There was a hell of a row about the missing money,' he recalled. 'Three of the patients had come back complaining they had definitely lost money while they were at the practice, and my partner reported his loss to the police. So we had irate patients at the desk, detectives asking questions, and the senior partner going around fully aware that I had something to do with the mess.'

Two loan-shark debts – incurred so he could clear the bookmakers' accounts – were soon collecting compound interest. Jonathan found it harder and harder to meet the instalments with enough cash to do more than clear that week's interest. He also found it hard to put up with the occasional threats, issued as timely warnings, which frightened him. He finally decided he must get money in larger quantities than he could from stealing – which, by then, was no longer a tenable proposition anyway.

'I couldn't help thinking while Jonathan was telling me about the new scheme,' said Dr Hibbert, 'that if he had expended even a quarter of that energy and intensity of purpose on his work, or on anything else productive, he would have been a highly successful man by now, a real brass-bound winner.'

Jonathan decided to start dealing in drugs. Several of his patients were addicts, and he had served on a drugs counselling service for a time, so he had a good idea of the price the various tablets, capsules and ampoules were fetching.

'We carried supplies at the surgery, though there was

only enough slack in the control system to allow me to take small amounts without raising suspicion. The way to really get decent quantities was with prescriptions.'

Using only his own prescriptions would not be a good idea, he decided, so he set out on a thieving mission, covering three associated surgeries in south London where he knew the partners and had reasonable cause to visit them. Over a period of four days he obtained nine prescription pads and stole a few from his own partners for good measure. Painstakingly he copied the doctors' signatures from specimens on various documents. For a time, he noted, the urge to gamble almost left him as he laboured to make the signatures look as close as possible to the originals.

'At the end of it all, around five o'clock one morning, I had several dozen signed blank prescriptions stacked on the table in front of me. They were potentially worth thousands of pounds. I was elated. I couldn't go to bed, I was so energised by the whole thing. I took a bath, shaved, changed into my best suit, then got into the car an hour before anyone was due to turn up at the practice. I just drove around London with a wad of prescriptions in my pocket, feeling bomb-proof, waiting for the chemists to open.'

That first morning he passed four forged prescriptions for barbiturates at chemists' shops in Piccadilly, Notting Hill, Fulham Broadway and Kensington High Street.

'I got the maximum possible on each and got a funny look or two in the process. Back in the car I sat and worked it out and estimated I could make two and a half grand with what I had.'

Dealing turned out to be harder than he had imagined. His face was unknown around the places where drugs changed hands, and wearing a business suit he realised he wasn't likely to attract inquiries. In the end, after spending two hours after morning surgery hanging about the West End with pockets full of barbiturates, he went back to the flat and changed into jeans and an old sweater. When he returned to the West End he found he could approach obvious-looking punters without frightening them away. Within an hour he had made six hundred pounds.

'And at that point,' said Dr Hibbert, 'the auto-destruct mechanism kicked in. He couldn't let himself win, after all. That isn't written into the program of pathological gambling. He had stolen prescriptions and obtained drugs and then obtained cash, all with a view to clearing himself of the entanglements of debt. So what did he do? He went to a betting shop and blew the whole six hundred quid in one afternoon.'

Afterwards, realising that he had done something profoundly stupid and self-damaging, Jonathan put more of the barbiturates into envelopes and went back to the vicinity of Greek Street, where he eventually made another hundred pounds, after narrowly escaping being reported to the police by an irate young man he had mistaken for an addict. Elated again, Jonathan went to a pub on Wardour Street that he especially liked, and he got drunk. In the course of the evening he kept buying drinks for other people as well as himself, and managed to spend the entire hundred pounds.

'Something very bad was happening to my personality,' he said. 'It was crumbling, and God knows it had got cracked enough by that time to crumble without much pressure.'

He went home and tried, for perhaps the first time in years, to evaluate his position and the state of himself as a human being.

'The same thing that was happening to me happens to prostitutes. They swear they'll work hard for a year and make enough money to retire, enough to get out of the business and live a clean life somewhere. And they mean it. But something happens, the very nature of what they do is so, I don't know, *unnatural* is the word that comes to mind, maybe it should be inhuman, or ugly, or gross or something like that ... Whatever it is, the life they lead gets to them and undermines their good intentions. They blow their money on stupid things – drinks, gaudy clothes to hide in, exotic pets, bloody huge teddy bears and other rubbish. They never save. You'll rarely ever meet one who has been able to save her money. And when you look at them you can see the ruination on their faces, the inner wreckage. I looked like that. I looked in the mirror and I saw it, the hopeless-whore face, the image of failure and self-destruction.'

The next afternoon, following surgery, he returned to the West End and sold more barbiturates. This time he went to the loan sharks and paid off some of his debt; at the last minute, however, he paid only half as much as he had intended, and took the rest to a betting shop, where he lost it inside two hours.

'In evaluating himself,' Dr Hibbert said, 'Jonathan thought he had put a rein on the dissipation, the breaking up of his personality. But all he had done was make a note of it, nothing more. In my view he wasn't capable of doing more than that. Without planning any further than the day and hour he was living in, he filled in more prescription forms and exchanged them for saleable drugs at chemists' shops all over London. He was working in the service of a hopeless cycle, and he tried not to listen to one small voice inside that was telling him it couldn't last.'

On the afternoon of the day he passed the second batch of prescriptions, he was sitting in the gardens at Soho Square, waiting to be approached by addicts, when two young black men came and dragged him to a car waiting by the gate. They pushed him inside, where a third youth hit him several times on the head and face with a leather sap, then took all the drugs and money Jonathan had on him.

Before they threw him out of the car again they warned him not to try selling drugs there again, or anywhere else in the West End. To drive home the warning they sat him against the railings outside the gardens and kicked him unconscious.

'I hadn't any clear idea how I got back to the practice, but I know I managed to drive there, and when I arrived there was a police car outside. Under other circumstances I would have been very cautious, but I was hurt, I was frankly despairing and I had this terrible unreasoning fear that I was going to die. So I walked straight in, without trying to detour up to the flat.'

The senior partner was standing in the reception area, talking to two policemen. They stopped talking when Jonathan entered. They stared at him. He realised he must have looked bad, in his old jeans and sweater, his eyes puffed half shut and dried blood all over his hands and face. One of the police officers was first to speak. He addressed Jonathan by name and told him he wanted him to accompany them to the station for questioning. In connection with what? Jonathan asked. Irregularities in connection with forged and stolen prescription pads, the officer said.

Jonathan was running back out of the building before he knew he had willed it. He hurled himself into his car, started it up and almost hit one of the policemen as he leapt at the passenger door.

'I drove like a crazy man,' Jonathan told Dr Hibbert. 'I probably *was* a crazy man. I was riding an imperative. I had to get away. Nothing else mattered or even existed.'

Incredibly, Jonathan did get away, and he managed to stay beyond the reach of the law for four months. But he was also, as Dr Hibbert pointed out, beyond the reach of any kind of hope or comfort. He had run away with nothing but his car. He did not have any money, anywhere to live, or even a change of clothes. For a time he managed to get bed and breakfast in a charity hostel, but was barred eventually because of his drinking. Unable to gamble any more – even when he had fifty pence to put on a horse, three different betting shops refused to take the bet and at one place he was literally thrown out – he turned to drink, most of it cheap cider, tonic wine or illicitly brewed 'electric soup' which sells for less than a pound a pint, and guarantees more than twelve hours of near oblivion.

'I tried, just once, to get in touch with my family. The response was incredible. Not only did my father shut the door in my face, but my brother threatened to get the police if I didn't clear off.'

Passing a shapeless succession of drunken days among derelicts living on the perimeter of Hyde Park, Jonathan lost any will to hang on to existence. At the time he was found and identified by a policewoman as she patrolled an underground car park, he had decided he would die. In his depleted state he believed that all he had to do was make the decision and it would happen. To keep out the cold while he waited, he drank tonic wine and any other alcohol he could lay hands on. A blood test taken shortly after his arrest indicated that another week of the wine-and-waiting regime would probably have granted him his release from life.

Dr Hibbert was keen to know how Jonathan felt now that he was on the way to being physically well again, and could accept that he had been suffering from a recognised mental disorder.

'I'm glad to be alive, and I think I'm making a good job of assessing what's been wrong and what needs to be done in the future. I've a feeling I'll be struck off the Medical Register, and I can't imagine anyone wanting to employ me when there are so many normal, fully-hinged individuals looking for jobs. Even so, I'm hopeful. I think I can turn out right.'

And what about the impulse to gamble?

'It's still there,' Jonathan said.

'Do you think you could give in to it again?'

He shrugged. 'I don't want to . . .'

Jonathan was eventually sentenced to two years' imprisonment, with the recommendation that he should receive therapy while serving his sentence. Dr Hibbert believed that given Jonathan's capacity for insight into his own condition, he might, with appropriate help, overthrow the 'need' element in his gambling impulse, and go on a support programme when he left prison.

The best support available at present is provided by Gamblers Anonymous, operating on lines closely similar to Alcoholics Anonymous. Local groups are run on an 'inspirational therapy' basis, with public confession, peer pressure and talks by reformed gamblers to help support the members' abstinence.

At the time of writing Jonathan has been out of prison for eight months and so far he has not relapsed. He is in a full-time job with a brush manufacturer and attends Gamblers Anonymous meetings twice a week. His suspension from the Medical Register is shortly to be reviewed and he hopes that if he stays firmly on the rails, he might return to medical practice within a year.

A Short Glossary
of Psychiatric Terms

Abreaction A release of suppressed emotions.

Acute Confusional State Damaged perception, judgement, reasoning, intuition, memory (the cognitive functions), with blurred, diminished consciousness. Can last for hours, days or even weeks.

Acute Dystonia Spasms of the neck, tongue and face muscles, usually as a side-effect of taking neuroleptics (q.v.).

Affect Emotion or mood.

Affective Flattening A noticeable lack of response to emotional stimulation.

Affective Incongruity Inappropriate emotional response, such as laughter at the news of a disaster.

Affective Personality Disorder A disorder marked by a tendency towards very noticeable mood swings. (*See also* Cyclothymic Personality.)

Affective Psychoses Disorders marked by mood disturbance ranging from deep depression to wild elation, with one or more of the following: delusions, hallucinations, pathological and unfounded guilt.

Agoraphobia A morbid fear of open spaces, with overwhelming anxiety, often leading to a panic attack.

Akathisia Uncontrollable restless movements in the legs caused by prolonged neuroleptic medication.

Ambivalence The simultaneous holding of two contradictory feelings or wishes.

Amnesia Loss or absence of memory.

Anhedonia A diminished capacity for experiencing pleasure.

Anorexia Lack of appetite.

Anorexia Nervosa A fear of putting on weight; food is rejected (not through lack of appetite); loss of 25% of body weight may occur.

Antisocial Personality Impulsive and aggressive, with no feeling for others, low tolerance of frustration, inability to accept restrictions imposed by law; behaviour not quickly altered by experience.

Anxiety Uneasiness in the mind; feelings of apprehension and fear.

Anxiety State Deep uneasiness and tension with vague pains and erratic, unintentional movements of the body.

Apraxia Inability to make deliberate movements, even though there is no physical illness or injury.

Asthenic Personality Tendency towards passiveness, with low energy and no capacity for enjoyment.

Autism A self-centred mental state; reality is excluded. (Infantile Autism is a psychotic disease that usually begins before the sufferer is three years old.)

Bipolar Illness Affective disorder with manic episodes, followed by episodes of depression. (Same as manic depression.)

Bulimia Bouts of extreme overeating followed by depression and self-induced vomiting, and/or purging and occasionally fasting.

Capgras Syndrome Delusions that people close to the patient are 'planted' doubles.

Catalepsy Trance with extreme body rigidity.

Catatonic Stupor	Silence and immobility seen occasionally in schizophrenia and Parkinson's disease.
Clouding of Consciousness	Impairment of consciousness showing reduced awareness of the surroundings and a loss of understanding of what is going on.
Cognition	Thinking, but used in psychiatry to mean memory and intellect as perceived in studies of mental states.
Cognitive	Perceptive, as a faculty rather than a feeling.
Cognitive Therapy	Treatments designed to change trends of abnormal thought which are believed to be the cause of some psychiatric disorders.
Compulsive Rituals	Things a patient feels compelled to do, often to a fixed and complicated schedule.
Concentration	The focusing of attention.
Confabulation	Manufacture of false recollection to fill gaps made by loss of memory.
Cyclothymic Personality	Personality typified by swings of mood from happiness to depression.
Déjà Vu	A new experience falsely perceived as a repetition. ('I've done this before'.)
Deliberate Self-Harm	*See* Parasuicide.

Delirium	*See* Acute Confusional State.
Delirium Tremens	A confusional state in alcoholics triggered by sudden withdrawal of alcohol; symptoms include tremor, restlessness, terror, hallucinations.
Delusion	False belief, quite impervious to reason, which is usually out of character for the patient.
Delusional Perception	The belief that an ordinary experience, object or event has important meaning for the patient.
Dementia	A persistent disorder of the mental processes marked by memory disorders and personality changes.
Denial	Rejection of reality to deflect unbearable experiences or thoughts.
Depersonalisation	Feeling of being unreal, or someone else.
Depressive Illness	A mental disorder marked by melancholy and other mental and physical symptoms.
Derealisation	Feeling that the surrounding world has become unreal.
Displacement	Shifting of distressing emotions to some other person, place or object.
Drug/Alcohol Dependence	A condition marked by compulsive drug or alcohol consumption to experience their

mental and physical effects, and often to evade the distress caused by the absence of the drug or alcohol from the system.

Dysarthria Defective speech.

Dysmnesia Impaired memory.

Dysmorphophobia A belief in one's own ugliness, in spite of a normal appearance.

Dsypareunia Painful sexual intercourse.

Dysphasia Impaired speech caused by a brain lesion.

Echolalia Parrot-like repetition of words spoken by others.

Echopraxia Imitation of another person's actions.

Ego The part of the mind which responds to reality and has a sense of individuality.

Electroconvulsive Therapy (ECT) Seizures induced by a current of electricity passed across the brain; used as a treatment in depressive psychosis.

Emotional Lability Instability of moods.

Empathy Identification with another person at a sound level of understanding.

Endogenous Originating from within a person.

Enuresis Bed-wetting.

Explosive Personality Disorder A chronic potential for angry or violent outbursts.

Extrovert Sociable, mainly concerned with

external matters or objective considerations.

Factitious Disorder Disorder that is not real, but is fabricated by an individual with a severe personality disorder.

Flight of Ideas A fragmentary stream of talk. Often found in extreme manic states.

Folie à Deux Simultaneous psychosis in two closely related individuals.

Formal Thought Disorder *See* Thought Disorder.

Formication A sensation like insects creeping on the skin. A common side-effect of cocaine withdrawal.

Ganser's Syndrome A factitious disorder in which the patient mimics, badly, the symptoms of psychosis.

Gilles de la Tourette's Syndrome Involuntary, purposeless movements, often with uncontrollable swearing and other taboo language.

Hallucination The alleged presence of an object or being that is not really there.

Hyperkinetic Syndrome of Childhood Disorder where a child has a short span of attention and is extremely physically overactive.

Hypnagogic Hallucination Hallucination which occurs in the moments between waking and sleeping.

Hypnosis Artificially induced sleep in which the subject acts on

	external suggestion.
Hypochondriasis	Abnormal anxiety about one's health.
Hysteria	A disturbance of the nervous system with psycho-neurotic origins, which can simulate the symptoms of almost any disease.
Ideas of Reference	An impression that other people's actions or conversation have reference to oneself.
Infantile Autism	(Same as Childhood Autism) A syndrome beginning before the age of three which is marked by social withdrawal, difficulty in understanding or using speech, and ritualistic behaviour.
Insight	A patient's awareness of his own mental condition.
Introvert	A personality type: shy, sensitive, inward looking.
Libido	The sexual drive.
Manic Depressive Psychosis	*See* Affective Psychoses.
Manic Illness	A disorder characterised by unusual elation.
Masochism	Sexual gratification derived from one's own pain or humiliation.
Morbid (Pathological) Jealousy	Delusion of a partner's infidelity in which the patient constantly searches for proof.
Münchausen's	Repeated attendances at

Syndrome	hospitals with spurious physical illness, often leading to drug treatment or surgery.
Münchausen's Syndrome by Proxy	A category of child abuse where adults (usually parents) give false histories of children's symptoms, and may fabricate the signs. Some children are known to collude in the faking of symptoms. Commonest signs reported are neurological, bleeding, and skin eruptions.
Negativism	Behaviour marked by patient not performing suggested act, often doing the opposite.
Neologism	The use of concocted words which may be meaningless – often a schizophrenic symptom.
Neuroleptics	Powerful drugs with anti-psychotic properties.
Neurosis	Any of a group of disorders with no physical basis, marked by anxiety, phobias, obsessive-compulsive behaviour and depression; contact with reality is maintained.
Obsessive-Compulsive Disorder	Repeated intrusive thoughts, impulses or actions which the patient knows are unreasonable and tries to resist.
Obsessional Personality	Perfectionist, unyielding, suspicious, prone to habitual checking.

Paranoia
Delusions of persecution and self-importance, with an abnormal tendency to mistrust others.

Paranoid Personality
Suspicious and emotionally hypersensitive, with a tendency to bear grudges.

Parasuicide
(Synonymous with Deliberate Self-Harm.) Deliberately non-fatal self-injury.

Perseveration
Repetition of a word or phrase, or repetition of answers unrelated to questions being asked.

Personality Disorders
Defects in temperament, general outlook on life and response to people and environment. *See* under separate headings.

Phobic State
Attacks of fear connected with aversion to certain objects or situations.

Pica
Eating substances which are not food.

Pick's Disease
Pre-senile dementia, occurring before the age of 65, with weakening of memory and unpleasant changes of personality.

Pressure of Speech
An onrushing flow of unusually rapid speech.

Primary Delusion
A belief with no discernible source, taking the form of

	absolute certainty that an ordinary, unexceptional event has great metaphorical meaning.
Projection	Putting the blame for one's own bad thoughts or impulses on other people.
Pseudocyesis	False pregnancy.
Psychiatry	The study and treatment of mental disorder.
Psychoanalysis	Methods of eliciting from patients their past emotional experiences and their part in influencing their present mental life, in order to discover the conflicts producing their disturbed or disordered mental state, and provide hints for therapeutic procedures. Psychoanalysis is also a system of theoretical psychology.
Psychology	The study of the human mind and its functions.
Psychometry	The measurement of mental abilities, using standardised tests.
Psychopathic Personality	*See* Sociopathic Personality.
Psychopathology	The scientific study of mental disorder.
Psychosis	Severe mental disorder marked by absence of insight and poor contact with reality.
Psychosomatic	The relationship between

mental and physical factors in illness.

Psychotherapy   Treatment of mental disorder using suggestion, persuasion, etc., to combat failure to cope with daily life and to encourage strengthening of personality.

Puerperal Psychoses   Psychoses occurring within three months of childbirth.

Rationalisation   Invention of reasons to account for personal inadequacy and render it palatable or acceptable.

Reaction Formation   Hiding unsavoury or antisocial thoughts or impulses by displaying opposite behaviour and expressing opposing ideas.

Regression   A return to immature, childish behaviour.

Repression   Shutting-out of unacceptable impulses, memories, etc.

Retardation   Slowness of speech and movement often seen in acute depression.

Sadism   Sexual pleasure derived from inflicting pain or humiliation.

Schizoaffective Illness   Psychosis combined with schizophrenic and manic or depressive symptoms.

Schizoid Personality   Diffident, retiring, emotionally cool, sometimes eccentric.

Schizophrenia   A group of related disorders, with disturbances of thinking, mood and behaviour. There is a characteristic sense of being controlled, and usually a range of delusions; diagnosis is difficult because of wide variations in symptoms.

Separation Anxiety Powerful fear of being separated from loved ones.

Sociopathic Personality Impetuous, belligerent, indifferent to others, easily frustrated, behaviour mostly unaltered by experience.

Stereotypy Repetitive actions – e.g. waving the arms, jerking from side to side, nodding sharply – which appear to be intentional, but have no purpose.

Stupor A condition of torpor or lethargy, with reduced responsiveness.

Tardive Dyskinesia Involuntary spasmodic movements of the tongue and facial muscles often caused by prolonged medication with neuroleptics.

Thought Block Typically, the patient suddenly stops talking and says his or her mind went completely blank, or empty.

Thought Broadcast A belief that one's thoughts can be heard by people nearby.

Thought Disorder Disturbed structure of continuous thought, with loosened associations; i.e. weak link between one idea and the next.

Thought Insertion   The conviction that alien thoughts are being planted in one's mind.

Thought Withdrawal   Belief that thoughts are being removed from one's mind.

Tic   A spasmodic contraction of the muscles, usually of the face.

Tourette's Syndrome   *See* Gilles de la Tourette's Syndrome.

Transference   A mental process whereby a patient transfers patterns of feelings and behaviour previously felt with important figures (parents, siblings) to another person. Often these feelings are transferred to the psychiatrist.

Trans-Sexualism   Firm belief that one is the wrong gender, with attendant desire for sex change.

Transvestism   Sexual pleasure derived from wearing clothes of the opposite sex.

Unipolar Illness   Affective disorder marked by recurring depression.

Further Reading

Bluglass, R, and Bowden, P. (1990) *Principles and Practice of Forensic Psychiatry.* Churchill Livingstone, London.

Brain, W. R. (1985) *Diseases of the Nervous System.* (9th edn) (revised by J. N. Walton). Oxford University Press, Oxford.

Culver, C. and Gert, B. (1982) *Philosophy in Medicine.* Oxford University Press, New York, USA.

Enoch, M. D. and Trethowan, W. H. (1991) *Uncommon Psychiatric Syndromes.* (3rd edn). Butterworth-Heinemann, London.

Ford, C. and Beach, F. (1951) *Patterns of Sexual Behaviour,* Harper & Row, New York, USA.

Freud, S. (1908) Morality and Nervous Illness: in *The Standard Edition of the Complete Psychological Works of Sigmund Freud, Vol. 9.* Hogarth Press, London.

Gelder, M., Gath, D. and Mayou, R. (1990) *Oxford Textbook of Psychiatry.* Oxford University Press, Oxford.

Gregory, R. L. (ed) (1987) *The Oxford Companion to the Mind.* Oxford University Press, Oxford.

Gross, R. D. (1990) *Psychology*. Hodder & Stoughton, London.

Inbau, R. E. and Reid, J. (1967) Criminal Interrogation and Confessions. (2nd edn). Williams & Wilkins, Baltimore, USA.

Kaplan, H. I. and Sadock, B. J. (1991) *Synopsis of Psychiatry*. Williams & Wilkins, Baltimore, USA.

Lyttle, J. (1988) *Mental Disorder*. Ballière Tindall, London.

McGarry, A. L. (1973) *Competence to Stand Trial & Mental Illness*. Rockville, Maryland, USA.

Rachman, S. and De Silva, P. (1980) *Obsessions and Compulsions*. Prentice-Hall, Herts.

Simmons, J. (1969) *Deviants*. Glendessary Press, New York, USA.

Spence, S. H. (1991) *Psychosexual Therapy*. Chapman & Hall, London.

Szasz, T. (1973) *The Manufacture of Madness*. Paladin, London.

Wing, J. and Creer, C. (1980) *Schizophrenia at Home*. National Schizophrenia Fellowship, London.

Winokur, G., Clayton, P. and Reich, T. (1969) *Manic-Depressive Illness*. C. V. Mosby, St. Louis, USA.

Young-Bruehl, E. (1990) *Freud on Women*. Hogarth Press, London.

Index

A selection of non-fiction from Headline

THE DRACULA SYNDROME	Richard Monaco & William Burt	£5.99 ☐
DEADLY JEALOUSY	Martin Fido	£5.99 ☐
WHITE COLLAR KILLERS	Frank Jones	£4.99 ☐
THE MURDER YEARBOOK 1994	Brian Lane	£5.99 ☐
THE PLAYFAIR CRICKET ANNUAL	Bill Frindall	£3.99 ☐
ROD STEWART	Stafford Hildred & Tim Ewbank	£5.99 ☐
THE JACK THE RIPPER A–Z	Paul Begg, Martin Fido & Keith Skinner	£7.99 ☐
THE *DAILY EXPRESS* HOW TO WIN ON THE HORSES	Danny Hall	£4.99 ☐
COUPLE SEXUAL AWARENESS	Barry & Emily McCarthy	£5.99 ☐
GRAPEVINE: THE COMPLETE WINEBUYERS HANDBOOK	Anthony Rose & Tim Atkins	£5.99 ☐
ROBERT LOUIS STEVENSON: DREAMS OF EXILE	Ian Bell	£7.99 ☐

All Headline books are available at your local bookshop or newsagent, or can be ordered direct from the publisher. Just tick the titles you want and fill in the form below. Prices and availability subject to change without notice.

Headline Book Publishing, Cash Sales Department, Bookpoint, 39 Milton Park, Abingdon, OXON, OX14 4TD, UK. If you have a credit card you may order by telephone – 0235 400400.

Please enclose a cheque or postal order made payable to Bookpoint Ltd to the value of the cover price and allow the following for postage and packing:
UK & BFPO: £1.00 for the first book, 50p for the second book and 30p for each additional book ordered up to a maximum charge of £3.00.
OVERSEAS & EIRE: £2.00 for the first book, £1.00 for the second book and 50p for each additional book.

Name ....

Address ....

....

....

If you would prefer to pay by credit card, please complete:
Please debit my Visa/Access/Diner's Card/American Express (delete as applicable) card no:

Signature .... Expiry Date ....